Dr Graham Easton is a practising GP, Fellow of the Royal College of General Practitioners and Programme Director for GP Speciality Training at Imperial College Medical School, where he trains medical students and junior doctors in general practice.

He has twenty years' experience as a successful communicator of medical ideas to the non-medical public. He was senior producer and presenter in the BBC Radio Science Unit, presenting Radio 4's *Case Notes* and a range of other programmes. He is a regular guest and occasional presenter on *Health Check*, the BBC's global health radio programme.

He was an editor at the *British Medical Journal* for four years and is on the editorial boards of the *British Journal of General Practice* and *Education for Primary Care*. He has had his own regular columns on the BBC Health website and for *Eve Magazine*. He is co-author of *How to Pass the CSA Exam* and *General Practice at a Glance* (first-prize winner in the Primary Care category at the BMA Book Awards 2013).

Praise for *The Appointment*

'A fascinating account of what it's actually like to be a GP dealing with all the surprises that come your way, appointment after appointment, in those ten minute slots they have to deal with all your ailments every morning. A very engrossing read.'
Jonathan Ross, *The Radio 2 Arts Show with Jonathan Ross*

"Buy it; read it; recommend it – *give* it, if necessary – to anyone who needs to be set straight about the worth and complexity of general practice."
Roger Neighbour, OBE, Past President of the Royal College of Practitioners

"This book should be available on prescription. . . This isn't a book simply for the 'interested lay reader': it is a book for anyone with an interest in medicine, from a sixth-former contemplating a career in medicine, a medical student wondering about general practice, a GP registrar struggling with the challenges of the consultation, a specialist trainee wondering what general practice is all about, and everyone in the NHS with a responsibility for primary care. It is a book for all patients and, of course, we are all patients".
Professor Roger Jones, Editor, *British Journal of General Practice*

"I really enjoyed *The Appointment*. I thought it was a well-written and easy-to-read book. . . It was a very honest and eye-opening account of a GP's day that made me both respect what GPs do and how much they have to know, but also made me sympathise with them more as human beings, not just diagnostic machines. . . I really enjoyed the book and I learned a lot from it and I would recommend it to anyone."
Ruth, *Radio 2 Book Club* listener

"I enjoyed the book tremendously. I found it engaging, interesting and enlightening! It also shows how much thought and care goes into looking after patients."
Anonymous, Patient

the
Appointment

Dr GRAHAM EASTON

ROBINSON

ROBINSON

First published in Great Britain in 2016 by Robinson

This paperback edition published in 2017 by Robinson

Important Note

You must not rely on the information in this book as an alternative to personal
medical advice from your doctor or other appropriate healthcare professional. You
should never delay seeking medical advice, disregard medical advice or discontinue
medical treatment because of what you read in this book. If you have any concerns
about your health, consult your doctor or other healthcare professional.

A CIP catalogue record for this book
is available from the British Library.

ISBN: 978-1-4721-3633-6

Typeset by Hewer Text UK Ltd., Edinburgh
Printed and bound in Great Britain by CPI Group (UK) Ltd, Croydon CR0 4YY

Papers used by Robinson are from well-managed forests
and other responsible sources

Robinson
An imprint of
Little, Brown Book Group
Carmelite House
50 Victoria Embankment
London EC4Y 0DZ

An Hachette UK Company
www.hachette.co.uk

www.littlebrown.co.uk

Dedicated to the memory of Dr John Easton

Contents

Preface

Twenty-five years ago, when people at a party discovered that I was a doctor, they'd usually ask me for a diagnosis or a recommendation. Things have changed. These days, people are much more likely to ask me to justify my medical thinking, or their own doctor's reasoning. The same is true in clinic encounters. Gone are the days of 'doctor knows best'. Right now we're redefining the relationship between doctor and patient, and for a relationship to flourish it needs to be built on trust, through openness and honesty. So in this book I'm opening up, with an intimate and honest account of what's going on in one GP's mind during a typical morning surgery (if such a thing exists).

The consultation is the central act of medicine, the heart of the relationship between doctor and patient. As a GP I have spent many years analysing, and teaching about, what goes on in those precious ten minutes. I still find it endlessly fascinating. Now it's time for patients to be let in through the consulting room door; this book, for the first time, makes that possible. You can join me on a real-time journey through a typical morning clinic of eighteen ten-minute appointments. Witness the vast range of problems that GPs have to tackle, just between breakfast and lunch. What it's like not knowing who or what will walk through the door next. I want to reveal the inner world of a modern GP as I navigate each consultation, from 'connecting' with you and getting the information I need, to spotting signs, making diagnoses, and deciding on the best tests and management. All this within the constraints of a ten-minute meeting in a health service stretched to breaking point.

I also want to shout from the rooftops about the vital role of expert medical generalism in an increasingly specialised profession. I am hugely proud to be a generalist, and every day I see the value in taking a whole-person view of health. Yes, I must think scientifically and analytically to make clinical diagnoses. But generalists don't just think of you as a body part that's gone wrong – we try to see the whole of you. Your family, your views, your history, your hopes, your worries. And we're with you for the whole journey from cradle to grave. With more people growing older, often living with several long-term conditions and lists of medications, someone needs to be keeping an eye on the big picture and helping you navigate through an increasingly complex health system. Someone needs to make sense of the unsorted health problems that don't fit neatly into one specialist silo or another. It's no wonder that countries all over the world still look to the UK to see how generalist medicine is done. Research in the UK, Europe and the US has shown that having more GPs or family doctors per head of population is linked to better health outcomes, cheaper services and a better patient experience. In a recent study of eleven rich nations the private, super-specialised healthcare system of the United States was judged the most inefficient. The independent Commonwealth Fund report found that although the US spends more than 17 per cent of its GDP on healthcare, it comes eleventh out of eleven on a range of health indicators. The UK primary care-based National Health Service (which spends about 9 per cent of GDP on healthcare) ranked first. Our much-maligned health service won top place on measures including effective care, safe care, access to care, coordinated care and patient-centred care. And yet primary healthcare, the cornerstone of the NHS and the envy of many countries without it, is under threat.

Although I'm writing from my doctor's perspective, patients are at the heart of everything. I want to be clear that the patients I see in this book are not real patients; out of respect for patient confidentiality I have created them all. But they are absolutely 'true to life'. They are characters and cases built up from twenty-five years of seeing real patients. The other professional colleagues mentioned in the book are also fictional (unless I've named them), as is the practice I describe. So if there's any close resemblance to any individual I have seen as a patient or otherwise, living or dead, it's entirely coincidental. I have called the patients by their initials (Mr DG, Master RC, Mrs CH and so on). That's sometimes how we talk about patients among the team, and it avoids the risk of me choosing a fictitious name which by chance belongs to a real patient. The initials are inspired by influential characters related to the case; I explain my thinking in the final chapter called 'Follow-up', which also gives a brief summary of what happened next with each patient.

In the few cases where I have told stories about real patients, I have asked for their express permission and have anonymised their details. I am hugely grateful to them for allowing me to include their stories in this book. On one or two occasions where I have not been able to ask permission directly from a patient, usually because they can't be traced, I have changed any recognisable details. The core truth of the story is still there, but the characters and most of the detail have completely changed.

Each case starts with the sort of medical summary I might see on the computer before a patient comes in. There's also a very brief background to what the patient is thinking before their appointment – though of course I am not privy to that insight in normal practice.

Although I have tried to make this fictional surgery as typical and authentic as I can, I do not presume to be speaking on behalf of all GPs. I can only give you a taste of how I think; what is on my mind. No two consultations are the same, and no two doctors will think about a case in exactly the same way. Nor do I pretend that what I present here is in any way a 'gold standard' of what should happen when you see your doctor. None of us is perfect, especially not me. The cases I describe reflect that. We know, for example, that up to 15 per cent of all medical cases are misdiagnosed, although most of the time (thank goodness) such errors don't lead to serious harm. I have done my utmost to ensure that the medical details are accurate and up to date and I have provided a list of key references for each chapter at the end of the book. I am extremely grateful to my experienced GP-trainer colleagues Dr Martin Block and Dr Neil Crowley, to Professor Azeem Majeed (concerning positive predictive values), to Professor Michael Coleman (concerning cancer survival statistics), to

Professor Paul Booton (in the chapter on headache) and to consultant urological surgeon Mr Justin Vale (in the chapter about the prostate cancer test) for checking that I am not way off the mark and haven't made any major medical 'howlers'. Having said that, any errors are my own and I take full responsibility for them.

I have enormous admiration for my GP colleagues. Because of my research and teaching, I only spend part of my week seeing patients. Most GPs work tirelessly, day in day out, face to face with their patients, helping, healing and managing risk. They are understaffed and overworked, micro-managed, super-scrutinised and often criticised. Funding for primary care is shrinking, patient expectations are rising, and workloads are ballooning. In a British Medical Association survey published in July 2015, over 70 per cent of GPs reported that their workload was unmanageable or unsustainable. The last thing they need is someone undermining them in any way. My intention here is the exact opposite; I want to show what a fascinating, complex, challenging and worthwhile job they do.

Getting Ready

My stomach fizzes as I fiddle with the keys to the surgery front door. Rattling keys and jangling nerves. It's an uneasy blend of anxiety and excitement, like pre-show tension for an actor. Sometimes I glimpse on the outside wall the brass plaque with my name and qualifications on it. That can be a boost, but just as often it makes me feel like an imposter.

All I know for certain is that for the next three hours or so, I will see at least eighteen patients. I have no idea what problems each will bring, or what skills or knowledge I'll need this morning. If I think too hard about it, it can seem overwhelming. I try to suppress any niggling worries about not knowing what to do, not being able to help. I shrug off intrusive images of missed diagnoses, sick children, collapsed patients, angry relatives, and an impossible mountain of demands and queries. I try to take a salami-slicing approach: when you're faced with a giant sausage, chop it up and tackle it one slice at a time. That way, everything seems more manageable. Sometimes I fantasise about what it would be like to have specialised in, say, the hand, or the eye, rather than the whole person. Then I could be pretty sure what's going to walk through the door each day. But I know I'd get bored with the same part of the body all the time. I like the challenge of a medical medley – the curriculum for GP training is pretty much 'anything'.

It's reassuring to see a friendly receptionist's face and I share a cheery 'morning' with the practice nurse (as cheery as is possible at 7 a.m.). I pop my head round the door of the doctor's in the room next to mine; even a few seconds' connection with a soul mate can charge me up for the morning. Although we're a team, a GP's job can be a solitary one.

Leabharlanna Fhine Gall

After saying our hellos and 'How are you doing?' we scuttle off to our separate hutches for the next four hours.

I notice a message in my pigeon-hole from one of the other doctors. 'Graham – FYI – Mr DG coming to see you today. PSA 105. Dr X.' A squirt of adrenaline makes my chest tingle and my fingertips buzz. I know Mr DG well. We get on; I like him. That blood test result means he's probably got prostate cancer. Out of the blue. Poor man. That's going to be a challenging conversation. I run through a brief internal rehearsal of how it might go.

My consulting room is, well, clinical. Two office-style wooden chairs with red material upholstery for patients, my desk with a black computer on it, and shelves with medical books and clinical paraphernalia. There's a whiff of alcohol rub and disinfectant. It's January, and my Velux windows look out onto a frosted wasteland of suburban back gardens; sheds, trampolines, old bikes and benches, all now draped in a silvery winter blanket. Because no one must look in, I pull down the blinds. The only nod to life outside is a photo of my wife and two children. It's a holiday snap from years ago, and they're all peering out through a hole in an ancient castle wall. That, and my drug-sponsored coffee-stained mug, are like time portals from science fiction; highways to calmer moments whenever things get too much.

I raise my swivel chair a few inches – I share this room with a part-time doctor, who is shorter than me. According to general-practice-training 'feng shui', we shouldn't have the desk between us and the patient, as a barrier. So I arrange the patients' chairs around the corner of the desk.

I gather my tools, like a knight preparing his trusty weapons and armour before battle. First, the Littmann stethoscope my father bought me when I qualified, black rubber and brushed metal. When I swivel the head from flat to bell, it makes a reassuring click like the smooth clunk of a luxury car door. It's the Mercedes of stethoscopes. I open my Keeler instrument set: ophthalmoscope (for looking at the back of eyes), otoscope (for looking in ears), and ear pieces – also with love from Dad (he was a doctor – a haematologist, a blood specialist. He had a go at general practice as a young man, but it didn't suit him. I think his initiation was during a crazy flu epidemic). I need my official practice stamp as well, and my tendon hammer and tuning fork. Then there's my pregnancy 'wheel' (a calculator for delivery dates), and another one to work out how hard asthmatics should be able to blow into a meter. Finally, a selection of vital leaflets, forms and protocols that I've collected into a box folder, all arranged alphabetically for quick access. The ones I really need to hand are my sick-note pad, and leaflets for referring people for counselling and physiotherapy. They go like hot cakes.

I'm wearing my GP uniform. My dad would be horrified by my suit-less and tie-less outfit; open-neck shirt, comfy jumper, everyday trousers. But my clothes are just an outward sign of an evolving doctor–patient relationship.

If I can remember all my passwords, and find my NHS smart card, I eventually access the surgery's computer records system. The first patient arrives at 7.30 a.m., so I have twenty minutes or so to tackle any test results, letters or queries that have arrived for me since yesterday. It feels good to clear the decks as far as possible before it all starts to mount up again.

I glance down the list of patients on my list so far. Several slots are held free until 8 a.m. so that, in theory, patients who need to see a doctor today can ring up and book an appointment. So until about 8.03 a.m., my list is not entirely full, but I can see who has booked already.

Some names leap off the screen. Some are 'frequent fliers'; I see Mr WE and Mr NA pretty often. Others are people with whom I have developed a close working relationship over the years, like Ms AW – I look forward to those. Some – today it's Mrs CH and Mr EK – are people I have asked to come back for review, so I'm curious to find out how they're getting on. Mr DG will be a tough one. Some names, I admit, make my heart sink. It's Mrs JI today. These are usually people with complex problems that I struggle with and who make me feel inadequate, some who save up lists of unconnected problems and expect them all to be dealt with in ten minutes, and just a few who can be extremely demanding or even rude. The rest are a mystery.

If there's time, I'll pick out a few names and brush up on the highlights of their medical history, or scan the most recent entry to bring

3

me up to date. I'll check if they need any health promotion or routine monitoring. In any case, if I forget, there's always a bossy pop-up window on the computer screen that shouts at me ('SMEAR NOT UP TO DATE'; 'ASTHMA ANNUAL REVIEW REQUIRED'; 'BP CHECK NEEDED'). That's partly about patient care, but primarily it's about getting paid. Like most NHS practices, we get paid a fixed amount based on the number of patients registered with us, but the rest (and this isn't a 'bonus' by the way, it's just how the practice gets paid) comes from payments for extra services (like special clinics), and 'performance'-related pay for meeting government targets on things like patient satisfaction, monitoring blood pressure and managing long-term conditions such as diabetes and asthma. Just doing the checks isn't enough though. To get your points, everything needs to be recorded using the correct code, the unique detailed template, the appropriate, endless, tick-boxes. In modern medicine, the computer is like a demanding gate-crasher in the room, barking orders, asking questions, bullying the consultation. An Aesculapian back-seat driver.*

Now it's 7.29 a.m. and my first patient has arrived. It says 'Waiting' next to his name. I still get that stomach-flutter of excitement and nausea I used to get before stepping onto the stage in a school play. But I feel more exposed and unsettled. Here, the cast keeps shifting and there's no script. Who – what – will walk through the door? Sore throat, meningitis, cancer, heart attack? Friendly, worried, furious, suicidal?

The curtain goes up and the performance begins.

* Aesculapius was the Roman god of medicine.

Chapter 1

Mr WE

`07:30`

Doctor view

Appointment time: 7.30
Name: Mr WE
Age: 33 years old
Occupation: Lawyer
Past medical history:
Tennis elbow
Medication:
None
Reminders:
Smoking cessation advice
Blood pressure check
Last consultation:
Two months ago, for sinusitis. It was treated with antibiotics.

Patient view

Mr WE is a 33-year-old lawyer who works long hours in the city. He's coping but he's been involved in an important deal recently which has been very stressful. He has come to the doctor because in the past few weeks he has been getting some sharp chest pains. The pain is fleeting and usually on the left side of his chest, where he imagines his heart to be. He has noticed that it's worse when he moves or when he takes deep breaths.

He tries to stay healthy. He drinks and smokes a bit – but only socially and he's not keen to cut down or quit at the moment. He goes to the gym five times a week and finds the treadmill helps him to wind down after a stressful day at work. He doesn't get any chest pain when he is on the treadmill. He has had the pain most days in the past month, and it comes and goes. He hasn't taken anything to help with.

Although he hasn't admitted it openly to his partner, he is worried that this pain could be coming from his heart – perhaps even a heart attack, as his father died of a heart attack aged 62.

I double-click on Mr WE's name and his records splash onto the screen. I've seen him a few times over the years, often with major concerns about minor complaints. A quick scan reminds me of multiple visits about normal male-pattern hair loss, niggling worries about his memory, and strings of tests for a nondescript skin rash. We've always got on well. He once told me that he likes how I don't judge him for his self-confessed health anxieties – his worried-wellness – and I admire his insight and honesty. He says things like 'I know it's probably nothing but . . .' or 'My partner thinks I'm a hypochondriac . . .'

I get up from my chair and walk down the short leaflet-lined passage that opens out into the waiting room. It's a chance to stretch my legs, and it feels friendlier than summoning patients to my room. Once I've called his name, any pre-surgery nerves vanish. Anticipation turns to action. I'm here now, in the spotlight with the patient, and everything else fades backstage.

He's lean; you might say stringy. His face is sharp, with bony cheeks highlighted by the cartoon shading of his beard shadow. There's his familiar intense frown, topped by thinning neat black, parted hair. I imagine those are his work clothes – pressed chinos, collared shirt, plain blue tie in a Windsor knot. He nods at me, with a brisk eyebrow signal, but keeps his eyes fixed on the floor as we walk back to my room.

'Morning. Come in, take a seat over here. How can I help you? I haven't seen you for a while.'

'Morning, yes. I'm fine thanks. It's a pretty straightforward problem actually. It's probably nothing . . . but I've been getting this chest pain, and I thought I'd better get it checked out. As I say, it may be nothing – you know I'm a worrier – but better safe than sorry.'

As he says 'chest pain', I pull the chest pain file from my medical memory bank. It contains hundreds, maybe thousands of cases, some from the hospital emergency department, some from general practice. There are a few lectures and chapters in there too, but it's the patients that really spring to mind. Most vivid are the heart attacks. Propped up on a trolley, grey and sweaty, heaving into a cardboard bowl. They can just about tell me through their groans that the pain's crushing them like a car on their chest, or squeezing like a tight giant chest-belt.

Maybe it's spread to their left arm or up to the jaw. They're often flabby, or smoky, and past middle age. Slim and youthful, pain-free and healthy pink, Mr WE clearly isn't in that bracket.

But he has the look of a frightened animal about him – perhaps he wonders if a heart attack might soon be his fate. The link between anxiety and chest pain is strong, but not straightforward. If you're anxious about your health, then your heart – the pump that keeps you alive after all – is a natural and common focus. But anxiety or panic attacks can also cause real chest pains; a sense of terror causes over-breathing, which in turn can upset the balance of oxygen and other chemicals in your body, leading to chest pain. Anxiety can also trigger genuine heart problems, and heart disease often causes anxiety. I have to keep all these possibilities in mind. And although it's often the heart that people associate with chest pain, I'm thinking of lots of other bits of him too.

So when he tells me that he has chest pain and describes it as a 'straightforward problem', I would disagree. In the next ten minutes I need to make sure that he doesn't have a potentially life-threatening cause for his chest pain that needs urgent attention, and, if I can elimi-nate those, work out what is wrong and what to do about it. But I'm not just hunting for a faulty part, like a car mechanic might. I need to deal with all of him, the whole complex, fascinating, flawed individ-ual. The worrier, the lover, the lawyer, the sufferer. That's a hell of a lot to cram into a ten-minute consultation. I don't want to start the morn-ing by getting behind, and there's very little room for error.

Only a fraction of the chest pain I see in primary care – about 8 per cent according to one study – comes from the heart. Most of it turns out to have a much more benign origin, like muscle aches and strains, indigestion with stomach acid flowing back up into the oesophagus (gullet), or anxiety attacks. In fact what flashes up in my head when someone mentions chest pain is a long list of possible causes, mostly minor, but a few extremely serious. I suppose I draw on a 3D image of the chest – the ribs and their contents like a bird cage stuffed with organs. The heart, yes, but also the two lungs wrapped around it like two hunks of purple bread round some pink heart-meat. The oesoph-agus, the stomach, and the main arteries are in there too.

I start out on a medical safari, on the look-out for the big game animals in chest pain. They're the predators I don't see often these days, but which I certainly don't want to miss. The king of the jungle is the heart attack, where part of the heart muscle dies through lack of oxygen from a strangled blood supply. Then there's angina – also caused by poor blood supply to the heart, but not yet damaging the muscle itself – another big beast. Then, deadly but easy to miss, there are serious lung conditions like a pneumothorax (a collapsed lung) or a pulmonary embolism (a blood clot that blocks the blood supply to the lungs). And the vicious killer I never forget (because one of my patients died from it many years ago when I was a trainee): a ruptured aortic aneurysm. This is where the main artery coming out of the heart – about the thickness of a garden hose – starts to bulge (an aneurysm) and the walls thin until they eventually burst. Few people survive.

My chief concern is missing one of these big game; sending someone home with a cheery 'it's not your heart', and hearing a few weeks later that they arrested in Sainsbury's. But I'm not so frightened of heart attacks or cardiac arrests in themselves. Like most doctors, I spent six months of my training as part of the cardiac arrest team in a hospital. To start with, as the rookie, whenever my arrest bleep went off I'd hold back a little to make sure my senior colleagues would get to the collapsed patient first. I felt it was in everyone's best interests. But as time went on, it became a familiar drill. By the end I may even have hoped to get there first, straddling and pounding chests, delivering electric shocks, injecting cardiac drugs. I even remember one snowy night when we all emerged from our on-call rooms in our surgical blues, racing with bleeps screeching to the wards across a sort of courtyard, and we all slipped over and landed in a giggling heap on the path. In the emergency department, the staple diet was managing heart attacks and angina – interpreting ECGs (heart tracings), giving pain relief, starting treatments. Admittedly, it's been a while since I've done all that frontline stuff, so it's a bit rusty – but it's pretty hardwired. And like all GPs, I have refresher training in resuscitation and life support every year, and I know how to get my hands on a defibrillator and some oxygen in a hurry.

Medical students are often told that 80 per cent of diagnoses are made on the basis of the patient's story alone, 5–10 per cent on the examination, and the remainder on investigations and tests. Whether the figures are accurate or not, they certainly feel about right to me. Chest pain is a great example: the key to getting the diagnosis right lies almost entirely in listening very carefully to the patient's story. So unless the patient is dangerously unwell and needs urgent treatment (and Mr WE doesn't have chest pain right now), it pays to take my time getting the story straight.

'Yes. Well don't worry – it may be nothing, but it's always wise to get chest pain checked out. So can you tell me more about the pain?'

Like all doctors, I've been trained to start the consultation with open questions – questions which can't be answered with a simple 'yes' or 'no'. The idea is that open questions will encourage the patient to tell their story in their own words, which gives us a richer, personal account. So, after Mr WE has delivered his opening comments (I'm aware that many patients rehearse their opening comments in the waiting room, or before, at home), I ask him something quite open, and then I shut up and listen. That doesn't mean just sitting there like a pudding, expressionless. Or looking at the computer screen. The modern GP is trained to be attentive, and to show interest by, for example, leaning forward, nodding, keeping appropriate eye contact or making encouraging noises like 'Right, I see . . .' or, 'Go on . . .', or, 'And was there anything else about it?' We call it active listening.

This isn't a rigid formula – every GP and every patient is different, so I have to choose the words or behaviours that seem comfortable and authentic for me, and for the patient in front of me. The key is to remain totally focused on the patient. In training we often practise these skills, testing out effective phrases and questions in simulated consultations with actors or colleagues, and by scrutinising videos of real consultations (with the patient's consent of course). Since the 1970s UK general practice has led the way in developing this deeper understanding of the doctor–patient encounter. The ten-minute consultation is the cornerstone of general practice, and what goes on in those precious ten minutes – how stories unfold, how events and relationships are shaped – is crucial to being an effective GP. If the surgeon's tool is his scalpel, and the radiologist's the X-ray – for a GP, it's consultation skills.

Actually it's more of a toolbox than a single tool. I pick and choose from a range of ingrained communication skills – body language, listening skills, turns of phrase, picking up on subtle cues. I might also draw on one of our many models of the consultation – imagine them as being like scaffolding to support the structure of a consultation, or a map to show me where to go. Things to do, and ways to do them. There's no single, unifying model of the consultation – we often borrow bits from different models and develop them over the years to develop our own individual consulting style. Before we're licensed as GPs, we're thoroughly tested on these skills – as well as clinical skills and knowledge – in a simulated surgery, each appointment being studied and scored by experienced examiners. I devoured books on consultation skills, went on courses, practised with friends; I was super-conscious of every non-verbal cue, every turn of phrase. But as the years go by, as with changing gear when I'm driving, I don't usually refer to the manual unless something goes badly wrong.

Mr WE seems anxious; his speech is pressured and his eye contact is not great. He looks at his lap. But he's responding well to my open questions and his replies are helpful and carefully considered.

'Well, they're quite sharp pains, just here.' He keeps pressing a point on the front of his chest over on the left side, below his nipple.

'Right, uh-huh,' I say, nodding encouragingly.

'It's when I take a deep breath it seems to get much worse, or if I move. I'll try to do the movement . . . it's when I do this.' He does an awkward squirm in his chair, like a clumsy slow-motion disco move.

'No, I can't quite get it now, but it's to do with moving shoulders or arms in a certain way.'

'OK, that's helpful. And is there anything else about it?'

This business of asking open questions and encouraging patients to talk is something that often bothers doctors. At medical school, we're taught the key questions to ask patients to help clinch diagnoses or rule out possible danger signs. These are usually closed questions with a restricted range of answers such as 'Where is the pain?' or 'Does the pain spread anywhere else?' For inexperienced medical students, or time-stressed doctors (I'll include myself), letting the patient 'ramble on' in their own words can sometimes feel like a waste of time. We're itching to get on and ask our key 'medical' questions before our ten minutes is up. In fact in one study, US researchers found that patients were allowed to finish their opening statement in less than a quarter of consultations, and that most doctors interrupted after about eighteen seconds. But, far from rambling on, the longest any patient took to complete their story was two and a half minutes, with most completed within forty-five seconds. And importantly, the study also found that patients often raised the most clinically significant concerns later in their story. A more recent study of UK GP consultations suggests we are doing better at listening these days: experienced GPs waited an average of fifty-one seconds before speaking (GPs in the first two years of training spoke sooner, at around thirty-six seconds). They rarely interrupted at all and mostly allowed their patients to complete their opening statements – which usually took less than a minute. So although I'm feeling the pressure of time – and may have one eye on the clock on my wall behind the patient – I try to shut up and listen for as long as I can. This is the golden minute (or two).

(***two minutes***)

Now I move on to what UK GPs like to call 'ICE'. This stands for the patient's Ideas, Concerns and Expectations. ICE is the Holy Trinity of consultation skills. It's such a central concept in general practice training that medical students and GP trainees often roll their eyes when trainers talk about it – they've heard it so often and it can seem fluffy to the more scientifically minded. It is the first step in an influential model of the consultation first proposed by Oxford-based social psychologist David Pendleton and his GP colleagues in 1984. But the reason we're still banging on about it is that people often come with their own ideas and worries about what their symptoms might represent, and about what they might be expecting or hoping for in terms of examinations, tests or treatments. If I never find out what your personal ideas, concerns and expectations are, then I simply won't be able to address your particular agenda and you may leave feeling unsatisfied or un-reassured, however smug I may be feeling about getting the diagnosis right. And with chest pain, in general practice, reassurance is often my most helpful offering.

Experience tells me that people have all sorts of ideas about their chest pain; they may be worried about a clot on the lung, or a muscle strain, or oesophageal cancer. Or they may not be worried at all – perhaps their partner sent them under sufferance. Perhaps they're just here for a sick note. So I need to give them the opportunity to tell me what's really on their mind.

Exploring someone's ICE without it backfiring takes some skill and experience. For a start, many patients don't have any sort of hidden agenda – they come simply because their throat hurts and they want it checked out. They haven't got any strong ideas about what it might be, and they're more than happy to hear what I think. By over-analysing a patient's reasons for coming I can easily put their hackles up. Another pitfall is taking the phrase 'Ideas, Concerns and Expectations' too literally. For example, I've heard doctors say things like: 'Do you have any ideas or concerns about what's going on here?', or 'And what were your expectations today?', or worse still, 'How were you expecting me to help you today?', which can sound dangerously sarcastic. If I get this wrong as a doctor, the answer to 'Do you have any ideas about what might be going on here?' is often, 'Well, you're the doctor – you tell me!'

Often alongside me in consultations – in spirit at least – is one of the gurus of GP consultation skills, GP and former president of the RCGP (Royal College of General Practitioners) Roger Neighbour (all UK GPs will have heard of him and his influential book *The Inner Consultation*, first published in 1987). He draws on several different disciplines to try to make sense of what goes on in consultations, including psychotherapy, communication skills theory and even sports psychology. His model has five main waypoints for the GP. The first is connecting: establishing a rapport with the patient. The second is summarising: working out why the patient has come, using skills to get at their ideas, concerns and expectations, and then summarising that back to the patient. Then comes handing over: the stage when doctor and patient negotiate a plan of action they're both happy with. Then there's safety-netting – making contingency plans for the worst-case scenario. Finally, and refreshingly, comes housekeeping: an acknowledgement of the importance of looking after yourself as a doctor, for the good of your patients. It's about clearing my mind of the psychological remains of the consultation so that I'm ready and raring to go for the next one.

I'm a big fan of Neighbour and his thinking. Reading his book was one of the most thrilling parts of my training. What really grabbed me was his description of useful skills to help achieve some of these waypoints. One example is a neat way to encourage patients to open up without making them feel stupid, and without making me, the doctor, look simple. He calls it 'My friend John' – a technique that introduces a fictional third party (he thinks of this as his 'friend John') into the consultation, to normalise health worries and make a patient feel more comfortable about revealing what's on their mind. So, instead of saying, 'Do you have any particular worries about what this might be?' I might say, 'I see a lot of people [my friend John] with chest pain who are worried that they might be having a heart attack. Is that something you're worried about?' The theory is that it's easier for you to admit to worrying about something when you know lots of other people worry about it too. Simple, but often effective.

'So WE, lots of people worry about chest pain and what might be causing it. I imagine you've already had some thoughts about that – or perhaps what we might need to do about it today? It really helps me to know whatever's on your mind before we go on.'

'Well, my father died quite young actually, from a heart attack. So obviously that is playing on my mind. I'm thinking I might need to get some tests done, maybe an ECG or something like that? Obviously you're the doctor – I'll go along with whatever you think is sensible . . .'

Nailing WE's ICE feels like a Eureka moment. As soon as I know what's on his mind, I'm halfway there. I still have my own medical agenda – I haven't been swayed from my tasks – but I am now much clearer about his. In the past, GPs were likely to stick pretty rigidly to their own medical agenda: thinking about the underlying pathology, looking for signs on examination, ordering investigations and planning treatments. It was the doctor doing stuff to the patient. The physician was in the driving seat. The danger was that I'd order an ECG and some blood tests to exclude any heart problems – and you'd go home still worrying it was a stomach ulcer. But GPs are now trained to take account of the patient's agenda as much as of their own and to come to a shared understanding of the problem and a shared plan of action. These days we're trying to be more 'patient-centred'.

It's great to hear a patient offering these precious ICE nuggets voluntarily at the start of a consultation, but in my experience this happens only rarely. Perhaps people are too worried about looking silly, or steering the doctor down the wrong path. Perhaps sometimes they are not even consciously aware of what's bothering them.

(*three minutes*)

I need to get on and ask some more of my medical-style questions. These are the questions we're taught at medical school: focused questions about the typical symptoms that go with specific illnesses. In particular, I need to rule out some of the big game in chest pain. It's a mix of sorting, sifting and sensing.

A good starting point is to enquire more deeply about the nature of the pain. Whenever a patient says they have pain – anywhere in the body – medical students have a set of questions they are taught to ask. One mnemonic that sometimes helps them to remember what to ask is SOCRATES. This stands for site, onset, character, radiation, associated symptoms, time course, exacerbating or relieving factors, and severity. (I recently discovered that some of today's super-bright medical students don't actually know who Socrates was. Nevertheless, they find the mnemonic invaluable.) So, for example, for onset, I ask when the pain came on and whether it came suddenly or gradually. Heart muscle pain often comes on gradually and gets steadily worse. And as for time course, serious heart pain tends to last more than fifteen minutes – less than thirty seconds is much more likely to stem from a non-cardiac cause. A fairly recent trend is to ask patients how severe a pain is by getting them to rate it on a scale of one to ten, where one is virtually no pain and ten is the worst pain they have ever experienced. It's a good way to get the patient's view of how bad it is, but I think the real attraction is that ascribing pain a numerical value offers a degree of comforting precision in an otherwise imprecise science.

For WE's chest pain, these SOCRATES questions are useful to rule out what's known as cardiac ischaemia – a lack of oxygen to the heart muscle. This relates to heart attacks or angina. If WE mentions certain symptoms in response to these questions, then potentially serious cardiac ischaemic pain is more likely. Fortunately his answers don't sound typical of serious cardiac chest pain. In particular, his pain doesn't come on or get worse with emotional stress or when he is exerting himself, getting better after a few minutes of rest (typical of angina).

'No, I don't get it when I'm in the gym on the treadmill. I can get it when I'm sitting on the sofa, or at my desk at work.'

It doesn't spread (radiate) to his arm or jaw. Nor does it sound like the typical crushing or squeezing central chest pain of a heart attack; his pain is sharp and fleeting and not too severe:

'It probably lasts a few seconds each time – maybe . . . five or ten seconds. It's a sharp stabbing sort of pain. How bad? Well, I suppose it's about 2 or 3 out of 10?'

It's usually on the left side of his chest – in fact he points to the exact spot on his ribcage. He doesn't feel ill in any way when he gets it (heart attacks often make people feel sick or sweaty, and there can be disturbances in the heart rhythm or breathlessness, too). A big clue is that he's noticed that it's worse when he moves or when he takes deep breaths. He's had the pain most days in the past month, and he's never had to take anything for it.

'So let me just check I've got this right. You've been getting some sharp chest pains in the past few weeks. The pain is usually on the left side of your chest, and you've noticed that it's worse when you move or when you take deep breaths. You feel it in the part of the chest just below your nipple there. And you're wondering whether it might be something to do with your heart, because your dad had heart problems, and you think you might need an ECG. Right?'

He responds with a curt 'Yup . . . yup', as if he's thinking, 'Come on, get on with it; we've been over this.' But I'd be taking a risk if I didn't at least do a quick recap at this point. For many patients, this summarising is a chance to correct or fine-tune the story. It's also about making sure I have understood him correctly before we move on.

As I say the words out loud, they start to tell me a medical story. Like the software on a dating site, my brain starts looking for a match from hundreds of cases of chest pain. My ears pricked up when he talked about it hurting when he takes a deep breath or makes certain movements. It's sounding very typical of pain coming from the chest wall – the muscles and soft tissues around the ribcage. If you strain muscles in that area, or have some inflammation of the rib joints, you will often find it gets worse when the ribcage expands or contracts (with breathing, coughing, sneezing or certain other movements), and you may well be able to point to a fairly specific area where you feel the pain. But I've also seen cases where pain on breathing is from the lining of the lungs (pleuritic pain) or from pericarditis (inflammation of the pericardium, the sac which surrounds the heart). These are both less likely, but potentially more serious. By listening carefully to WE's story and encouraging him to open up, he's pretty much told me the diagnosis already, as well as what we need to address in terms of next steps.

'That's it, doctor. I mean, if you don't think I need an ECG, that's fine – it's literally just an idea.'

(*five minutes*)

I'm starting to relax a bit. Some of the other possible causes of chest pain that I started out with in my head are fading away. I am much less worried now about, for instance, pericarditis, oesophageal reflux (stomach contents flowing back up into the gullet) or aortic dissection (a swelling of the main blood vessel in the body which starts to split open). Oesophageal reflux tends to be a burning sensation, rising up from the stomach or lower chest. It may be linked to eating, being overweight, lying down, stooping or straining, and it's usually relieved by anti-acid medication like, for example, Rennie's or Gaviscon.

The classic features of a panic attack are over-breathing, numbness or tingling in the fingers or around the mouth, and it can also make people feel light-headed, sweaty or dizzy. No mention of those. Pericarditis often gives a sharp stabbing pain that is worse on lying down and better when sitting up or leaning forwards. It does, though, tend to get worse on breathing in or coughing, so I haven't completely crossed that off my list yet. I also need to rule out pleuritic chest pain (chest pain coming from the lining of the lungs or 'pleura', sometimes caused by pneumonia or a clot on the lungs), which can cause a stabbing-type pain on taking a deep breath in. So I ask in more detail whether he has some of the associated features of pleuritic pain, such as a cough, breathlessness, or blood in his spit. Negative.

Some people are more at risk of heart disease than others. The evidence on this is very clear. So the next important piece of the puzzle is an assessment of WE's risk of serious cardiac disease – I need to give my hunches and theories some background context. If I spot something large and cat-like in a game park in Africa, it's probably a lion, a cheetah, or maybe an African wild cat. But if it's in my local park in West London, it's likely to be just a large pussy cat. I need to know what sort of park we're in.

I know his dad had a heart attack when he was young. I also ask whether there's anyone else in his family who's been affected, or if there have been any strokes, blood clotting disorders, or blood pressure problems. He doesn't have diabetes or high blood pressure. The strain on obese people's hearts puts them at risk, as does the laziness of un-exercised hearts. My computer can quantify someone's risky habits and history in terms of a number. At the press of a button I can estimate their risk of having a heart attack or stroke in the next ten years – a percentage risk score flashes up on the corner of my screen.

Anything above around a 10 per cent risk over the next ten years starts to ring alarm bells. The numbers help, but they're just an estimate, based on things like cholesterol, BMI (Body Mass Index, a measure of whether you're a healthy weight for your height), and whether or not one smokes or has diabetes. It's easy to treat the number and not the person. Most GPs I know would agree that we can often spot many of the high-risk patients as they walk through the door. The overweight older males who smoke and do very little physical exercise are at particular risk. WE is young and fit, with a risk score of only 2 per cent, but he has a family history of heart disease, his father having been in his mid-sixties when he suffered a fatal heart attack.

I need to ask some potentially sensitive personal questions about lifestyle to gauge WE's risk – smoking, drinking and exercise for example. It often helps to use a technique called 'signposting' – simply telling the patient what I'd like to ask about next and why.

'Thank you. Can I ask you some questions about your general health? Some of them are about smoking and alcohol – but they're just routine questions we ask everyone. Is that OK?'

This may seem rather basic or even unnecessary, but without this signposting of a change of direction in questioning, it's very easy to surprise or shock people, for example when changing gear from comfortable questions about their mouth ulcers to the intimate details of their sexual history (which could potentially be connected): 'So, you've had some painful mouth ulcers for about four weeks which don't seem to be going away. And have you noticed any sores on your penis?'

Mr WE tries to stay healthy. He drinks and smokes a bit, but only 'socially', he says (I should certainly pin him down on what that means exactly – we know patients tend to underestimate their drinking and smoking habits for the doctor – though I need to pick my moment). I ask him if he's keen to cut down or quit at the moment – he's not. I throw a titbit to the hungry computer, a special code for 'smoking cessation advice' – it will be counted towards our income. It takes me a while to find the code, but at least it stops the computer flashing at me.

WE goes to the gym five times a week. There's nothing of significance in his past history. So here's a young man who takes a lot of exercise, has no significant personal history of heart problems, and has no features of cardiac-sounding chest pain. There is a significant family history though, with his father's early heart attack. The picture is emerging . . .

It's always worth asking about medications, too; it often gives me a neat summary of a patient's main medical problems. People with lots of medical problems may not remember to mention that they have high blood pressure, but they will usually remember that they take a blood pressure pill every morning. WE isn't taking any medications, either prescribed or over-the-counter.

(***six minutes***)

I need to move on to examining him now. If I'm honest, I know that listening to his chest with my stethoscope is unlikely to help me much in terms of pinpointing a diagnosis. I won't, for example, be able to hear if he has a blocked coronary artery, or if he has an aortic aneurysm. But however confident I am feeling so far about what's going on, and however rushed I am, I can't afford to cut corners.

My stethoscope can pick up some of the echoes of heart disease that might accompany chest pain. I don't want to miss aortic stenosis (narrowing of the main outlet valve of the heart, which can cause angina – you can hear the change in blood flow due to the narrowing) or heart failure (a damaged heart doesn't pump effectively, so I might hear evidence of fluid building up in the lungs – a sort of crackling sound at the bottom of the ribcage at the back when one breathes in). Modern ten-minute medicine is often about playing safe: we're trained to exclude serious problems. But if it isn't life-threatening, pinpointing what the actual problem is can be a bit of an afterthought in medical education.

But before I get as far as laying a stethoscope on WE's chest, I need to look at him closely. Doctors call this 'inspection' – we're all taught to look first, before touching. The order is always:

1. Inspection (looking – generally, and then more closely).
2. Palpation (touching, feeling, for example the abdomen).
3. Auscultation (a fancy name for listening with a stethoscope).

Doing this in the wrong order in medical final exams risks failure. I'm not sure quite why the profession feels so strongly about this, but it's certainly true that the danger of diving in with a stethoscope is that you can miss the wood for the trees. Taking it in stages is a bit like zooming in slowly from a wide shot to the close-up. That way you're unlikely to miss anything. If you zoom in straight away, it's embarrassingly easy, for instance, not to notice that someone is as pale as whitewash or that they have the tell-tale scar of kidney removal hidden on their side.

I'm looking out for obvious signs of chest disease. WE is comfortable, not struggling for breath, and doesn't have the blueness of cyanosis around his lips or fingertips, which would be a sign that oxygen levels are dangerously low. I gently pull down his bottom eyelid, checking for the pallid pinkness of anaemia. I look to see if he has any xanthelasma (yellowy deposits in the skin around the eyes, which can be a sign of high cholesterol). Nothing.

I zoom in on his hands. Your hands are stuffed with medical clues. There are more health clues per square inch of your hands than anywhere else on your body, including your face. One of the most striking things I might spot in WE is finger clubbing. This is where the soft tissue around the ends of your fingers and toes increases and your fingers end up looking like matchsticks with a sort of clubbed end. No one really knows why it happens, but it can be associated with a range of conditions, from serious heart and lung disease to liver cirrhosis or inflammatory bowel diseases. More common is nicotine staining on the fingers – a giveaway for smokers. You may say you're not smoking any more, but your yellow-brown fingers will betray you. No sign. I check for little bleeds under his nails, like tiny splinters; sometimes a sign of infection of the heart valves. At medical school it feels like the most important sign there is – after years of real practice I don't think I've ever seen a case.

Mr WE doesn't notice me checking all these things. I've checked them out as he walked in, while I listen to his story, or with a quick glance at his hands and face while I'm tuned in to his chest. In medical exams, on the other hand, we are taught to make it very obvious to an examiner that we are looking for a specific sign – a bit like the exaggerated glance in your rear-view mirror for the benefit of your driving test examiner.

WE notices me checking his pulse though. I gently compress his radial artery against the underlying wrist bone; my fingertips now delicate heart sensors. No sign of the chaotic rhythm of atrial fibrillation, the frantic gallop of tachycardia, or the funereal pace of complete heart block.

I look closely at his neck and check for swelling in his ankles. With experience, the right lighting and a bit of luck, you can use the jugular vein as a sort of barometer of the pressure in the heart; the higher you can see it in the neck, the greater the pressure. Swollen ankles are much easier to spot. I press just above the ankle bone, checking for any indentation, like fingerprints in fresh dough. Ankle swelling or swelling of other parts of the body where fluid might collect due to gravity (such as the lower back when sitting or lying in bed) can be another sign that the heart may not be pumping as it should – not getting blood back to the heart. Again, there's nothing.

Now, finally, I can feel or 'palpate' his chest, and use my stethoscope to listen to his heart and lungs. Like most doctors, I have a close relationship with my stethoscope. Over the years I have come to think of it as an extension of myself, a trusted friend, and a kind of comfort blanket all rolled into one. Symbolically it's a kind of link between doctors and patients – an umbilical cord going from one to the other. It's often the only time we are physically connected to a patient during a consultation; a demonstration of thoughtful caring, which can be very powerful in healing. It's also a badge of honour – an icon of doctoring. But it's not a state-of-the-art diagnostic tool. I could probably hear your heart and lungs just as well by putting my ear against your chest (in fact the stethoscope was originally invented in 1816 by a French physician called René Laennec to listen to his overweight female patients without the embarrassment of getting too close to them by putting his ear against their bosoms). Patients seem reassured by the feel of metal on skin. It makes doctors feel like doctors too. I once heard a story from a colleague about a trainee doctor who went on a home visit but forgot his stethoscope. He'd already decided his patient needed antibiotics, just from her symptoms, but not wanting to disappoint his elderly patient, he took a coin from his pocket and pretended to listen at her back by pressing it against her skin and asking her to breathe in and out. It was all going so well until he realised that she was watching him in her dressing table mirror. 'Ah,' he said, quick as a flash, 'I'm just doing the special coin test.' Apparently he got away with it.

With my earpieces inserted, I am lost in a hypnotic cardiac symphony. It's usually the 'Lub-Dup' base beat of the valves opening and closing like a finely tuned engine. But sometimes there are the unusual whooshing or swishing sounds (heart murmurs) from the turbulent blood flow across leaky valves, or unexpected extra sounds, like clicks, from diseased or scarred valves opening and closing. If your mitral valve is leaking, Lub-Dup becomes Lub – shhhhh – dup. If you have a leaky aortic valve, it's Lub-Dup – shhh. I use both sides of the stethoscope's chest piece: the flat diaphragm is good for listening to high-pitched sounds such as lung wheezes, whereas the bell-shaped side is used for listening to low-pitched sounds such as grumbling heart murmurs from the mitral valve.

These heart noises are often painfully subtle: as medical students we often say we can hear them when we can't, to avoid looking stupid. With experience, you can hear them more easily, but even if you can hear a murmur, working out which valve is the problem can be extremely challenging, because there are four main valves all opening and closing at slightly different times. No wonder that when I was at medical school, one of our clinical tutors (a highly respected clinician) called stethoscopes 'guessing tubes'. It seemed spot-on to us. Fortunately, in recent years we have been able to turn to echocardiograms (which scan the heart while it's moving) to pinpoint valve problems much more accurately. This has been great for patients, but it has meant that nowadays we doctors are not as skilled as we were twenty or thirty years ago at diagnosing heart problems using a stethoscope – we just don't need to be. Nevertheless I am feeling confident that

WE doesn't have any major heart murmurs. But this is much more about excluding serious conditions – I'm not really expecting it to help me work out what's actually wrong.

Heart done, lungs next. I listen carefully over all the main lung zones, hovering in each spot while WE breathes in and out, and I compare one side with another – that way, any changes become more obvious.

'Breathe in and out through your open mouth please.'

I tune in to see if I can detect a different set of sounds now, mainly wheezes (the high-pitched squeaky noises you get in asthma or sometimes an infection) or crackles (as if someone is rustling a paper bag, which often suggests infection). I'm not expecting to hear anything in WE: this is mostly to reassure him that I am being thorough and to reassure myself that I haven't missed anything obvious like pneumonia. So I can usually complete these checks pretty quickly – though not through a thick jumper or even a shirt, as the material muffles any chest sounds and often makes its own crackling noises. (If your doctor regularly listens through thick clothing, I'd probably look for another one.)

If everything sounds normal, and if the history doesn't ring any alarm bells, having a stethoscope stuffed into my ears can be the cue for welcome peaceful reflection. I think about what's going on, piecing together the clues from the story and the examination. I gather my thoughts about my next steps in terms of management – pills, tests, advice, referral? My mind wanders to holiday memories – a glance at my family photo. I'm thinking about Mr DG and his prostate result too. What will I say? How will he take it? I snap out of my daydream and remember that WE is waiting expectantly to hear what I've heard.

'Well that all sounds completely normal,' I say with a smile.

'OK, great.' His eyes follow me, as if looking for tell-tale clues about what I'm really thinking.

'Yes – your heart sounds fine, lungs are all clear. So that's good news. Can I just measure your blood pressure, and then we're all done?'

In the old days, only I would know what your blood pressure was because it was measured using a mercury manometer while I listened to your pulse using a stethoscope. Only I could tell when your pulse was audible, and when it disappeared again – corresponding to the higher (systolic) and the lower (diastolic) numbers. It was my secret. That meant it was very tempting to say it was 'fine' when it was a little raised but not worryingly so – a white lie I'm sure many doctors told. But now we use digital machines that broadcast your blood pressure for all to see, so there's no room for 'fudging it' to avoid unnecessary worry. The way we record blood pressure – one number over another, 120/80 for example – is really just a measure of the maximum and minimum pressures in the circulatory system, no different from your central heating really. The higher number correlates to the highest pressure, as the heart pumps blood round with great force, and the lower number is a measure of the pressure in the system as the heart relaxes and refills with blood. Fortunately WE's blood pressure is well within normal limits today (128/80 – the normal upper limit for most of us is 140/90).

Normality is reassuring for him, and me, but doesn't really help to pinpoint the problem. My working hypothesis is still mostly based on his story; this is likely to be a chest wall problem (affecting the muscles or joints in the chest) rather than a heart or lung problem. Now time for a make-or-break test for my theory. I'm hoping that he may have some tenderness (the exclusive medical jargon for 'sore when pressed') when I poke him firmly in a specific area on the surface of his chest, or pain when he makes certain movements using the muscles and joints in the chest wall, or his arms. That would certainly support my thesis.

I gently prod systematically across his chest wall, especially around the area of cartilage which joins the ribs to the breastbone (sternum).

'Ow! Yes that's really sore actually.' His face screws up when I press over one or two of the joints near his nipple. I apologise for causing any discomfort, but inside I'm high-fiving myself for finding the final piece of the jigsaw.

'Sorry – didn't mean to hurt you. Is that the same sort of pain you've been getting?' I ask hopefully, trying not to lead him on too much.

'Yup, that's it – really sharp,' he says.

If this was pain from the heart, or from the lungs, it would be very unlikely that I could reproduce it simply by pressing on the chest wall. Things are really hanging together nicely now. It's time to wrap things up.

(*seven minutes*)

I'm glad I took the trouble earlier to establish WE's main ideas, concerns and expectations; I am now in a position to address his agenda straight on. The two key tasks in my mind now are: coming up with a clear plan of action with which both of us are happy (a double act between patient and doctor) and making sure I make clear what he should do if things don't go according to my predictions (preparing for the worst-case scenario).

'So, your symptoms, along with my examination, point very clearly to a problem with the chest wall which is causing your pains. I think you have a condition called costochondritis – literally, inflammation of the joint between the rib and the breastbone or sternum. Have you heard of that?'

'No, not at all.'

'Well, it can be very painful, and it tends to get worse when you take a deep breath or make movements with your chest. It's not serious though and it usually settles on its own over a few weeks – sometimes months. You can use anti-inflammatory medication like ibuprofen for the pain and inflammation, as long as there's no reason why you can't take those sorts of medicines.'

I'm scanning his face – he's nodding thoughtfully, encouragingly for me. I think this is making sense for him.

'So what could have brought that on then? I haven't injured it or anything . . . I think I would have noticed.'

'Well, it's not always possible to find out exactly what triggered it, but sometimes it's from an injury to the chest wall, strenuous lifting, even vigorous coughing. Sometimes from doing some kind of activity that you're not used to – like decorating or moving heavy furniture for example.'

'Well, I was helping a friend move some heavy furniture a few weeks ago, so I suppose it could have been that?'

'That's certainly the sort of thing that might trigger it. So the good news is that it doesn't sound at all typical of heart pain – even taking into account your family history of heart attack in your father. And your symptoms are so typical of this other condition that there's a case for not doing an ECG heart tracing because it's very unlikely to offer us any really useful information. But given your family history, it might be a good idea to do one anyway, just as routine. And we could check your cholesterol and blood sugar too, as a general heart health check. We haven't done that for a while. What do you think?'

'Yes, I think that's a good idea. Just to be on the safe side, you know. My partner's been nagging me to get it checked out, so she'll be pleased too!'

What I'm trying to do is frame my explanation of what's happening in terms that relate to his original agenda. I'm also checking that he is happy with my explanation, and I've deliberately left the door open for him to ask me questions or voice any concerns. I missed the pressure from his partner to get it checked.

I finish with what's called 'safety-netting' (another term coined by Neighbour): anticipating the worst-case scenario. I may have a pretty good idea of what's going on, or more importantly what's not going on (a life-threatening cause for his pain), but I always need to make sure the patient knows what to do if things don't turn out as I have predicted. In this case my safety-net involves telling him what I expect will happen: that things will gradually settle down with anti-inflammatories and laying off heavy gym work. Over a few weeks, there should be a noticeable improvement. But I also need to explain that if this doesn't happen – if things don't improve, or if they get worse – he needs to come back and see one of us. I also paint him a picture of a typical heart attack so he knows what symptoms to look out for, and I tell him that if he ever experiences these, he should go straight to A&E.

'OK? Does that all make sense?' I say with a 'we've come to the end now' tone of voice.

'Yes, Doctor. Thanks, that's a relief. I'm sorry for bothering you over nothing.'

'No – you haven't bothered me at all. It's important to get that sort of thing checked out. I think we've talked before, haven't we, about how you feel you worry unnecessarily about your health? I don't think that's the case this time – but is there any reason why this has surfaced now, do you think?'

'Well, no, it was really just thinking about my dad and his heart attack, you know.'

'Nothing else stressing you out at the moment?'

'No more than usual! Busy job of course. No, nothing really.'

'OK. Well, I'm always happy to talk that stuff through if you think it would help. Good. I hope this has been helpful. If you get those blood tests and ECG done and then perhaps we could meet after that to talk them through?'

I get up from my chair, a signal that we've finished, and we shake hands.

'Thanks for coming.'

'Yes, thanks. That all makes sense. And I'll see you after the tests.'

I can tell from his face – relaxed, with upturned mouth corners now – that we've hit the jackpot. Sometimes it feels like my job is really about shouldering other people's worries. The uncertainty is still there; like energy, you can't create it or destroy it – it's just been transferred from one of us to the other. It's as if, as he leaves free from his heart-shaped anxieties, he dumps all the unknowns, the risks and the dark cardiac possibilities, onto me. But this time, that burden is light – I'm as sure as I can be that his symptoms are not coming from his heart.

The computer is hungry again. It wants his blood pressure measurement, in the right box, in the specified format. It's a fussy eater. After I've written my notes, I fill in the template to make it shut up, and collect the points.

(**ten minutes**)

Chapter 2

Mr NB

Doctor view

Appointment time: 7.40
Name: Mr NB
Age: 36 years old
Occupation: IT manager
Past medical history:
Asthma
High cholesterol
High blood pressure
Medication:
Salbutamol inhaler (for asthma)
ACE inhibitor (blood pressure medication)
Reminders:
Needs blood pressure check
Needs cholesterol check
Consider starting cholesterol medication (statin)
Last consultation:
A year ago, for asthma

Patient view

Mr NB has noticed some blood on the toilet paper when he opens his bowels. It's happened three times in the last two weeks. His bottom has been a bit sore and itchy. He's terrified it might be cancer. He has seen adverts on the TV recently about the importance of getting blood in the faeces checked out. He has looked up his symptoms on the internet and thinks he probably has bowel cancer. He used to smoke, and his father died of kidney cancer aged sixty.

He knows he's likely to be examined with a finger in his bottom and he's concerned that he might break wind, or worse, during the examination. Part of him doesn't want to know the bad news – but on balance he'd rather find out what the problem is. His wife has also encouraged him to make an appointment.

Mr NB is new to me. I see that another doctor saw him for his asthma about a year ago, but he is not what we'd call a 'frequent flier'. In fact he's someone we'd like to see more often – to check his high blood pressure and cholesterol, both risk factors for heart disease. At thirty-six, he's at an age where I can imagine yellow fatty deposits starting to build up inside his coronary arteries. The computer is also nagging me to check his blood pressure today, and organise a blood test for his cholesterol. So I need to make the most of this rare visit to the surgery. This means two things for me: one, it's going to take longer, and two, I'll have to impose my own (actually, the computer's) agenda somehow on his appointment, which can feel rather autocratic. I get up and wander down the short corridor.

'Mr NB?'

He's big. The underlying frame is sturdy, a former rugby player perhaps, but now in middle age there's definitely some bonus bulk attached. He has to heave himself up from the brown NHS faux-leather banquette. He has a friendly, rounded face but he doesn't return my smile. I've learned not to judge people on these first impressions – doctors' waiting rooms breed all sorts of anxieties and vulnerabilities. But it does make me curious about what's on his mind.

'I'm Graham Easton,' I announce, with a not-too-jolly smile. I try to predict whether people want to hear 'Dr Easton', or the more informal 'Graham Easton'. It's not an exact science – I usually base it on age, and the gravity of the patient's facial expression – and I'm sure I don't always get it right.

'Hello,' he says. We shake hands.

'Come in, take a seat.' I shut the door behind us. 'So, how can I help today?'

I've dabbled with a few opening lines over the years. I've tried 'How are you today?', 'What can I do for you today?' and even the old favourite 'What seems to be the problem?' None of them feel quite right. They're all polite and friendly enough, but they can also dominate a patient's first thoughts. Even 'So, how can I help today?' has backfired on me, with a baffled response: 'Oh. How can you *help* me? I hadn't thought about that. I'm not even sure anyone can help me actually . . .' Patients have often prepared their opening lines – I know I do when I see the doctor. So it's much better really to hand control over to the patient completely and let them tell their story in their own words, without steering it in my direction. One way to do this is just to say 'Hello, nice to see you. Come in and take a seat.' Then, with enough non-verbal encouragement like a warm smile or a faintly raised brow, most people kick things off in their own words. 'How can I help today?' seems to have worked OK this time though.

'Well, it's a bit embarrassing actually.'

'OK, don't worry – go on . . .'

I shut up. David Haslam, a former Chair of the Royal College of General Practitioners (RCGP), neatly summed up the four key skills for effective consulting as: shut up; listen; know some medicine; care. That pretty much captures all the consultation skills we pore over and rehearse in great detail during our GP training.

I empathise with his embarrassment. I understand why people would rather look up their symptoms on the internet – or just stick their head in the sand – than have me scrutinise their private parts. But it can be a risky strategy. When I was a 14-year-old boy, my breasts started to grow. To me there were only two diagnostic possibilities. The first was too grim to contemplate: breast cancer. The second was too embarrassing for words: I was turning into a woman. I couldn't see how the school doctor could do anything other than confirm my worst fears or laugh at me; or both. Somehow my dad (a consultant haematologist) persuaded me to see the GP. After a solemn prod he confirmed that I had what's known as pubertal gynaecomastia – transient swelling of one or both breasts caused by the hormonal storm of puberty. It's normal and affects about half of all boys at that stage. He was calm, understanding, kind, and not at all patronising. Instantly my changing-room phobia and D-cup anxieties melted away.

If the internet had existed in those days, I'd have gone surfing. If I had Googled 'breast swelling in boys' I might have come up with gynaecomastia and breathed a huge sigh of relief. But if I had typed in 'lump in breast' or 'male breast cancer' it might have been a very different story. I would probably have been what we now call a 'cyberchondriac'. Either way, my best bet was to get properly checked out by someone with the experience (and kindness) to assess my particular problem and put it into some kind of perspective.

'Well, over the last couple of weeks or so, I've had some blood when I go to the loo. Maybe two or three times. So . . .'

He leaves his 'so' hanging for longer than I was expecting. I realise that he's not planning on saying anything else just yet. It's as if he has delivered his bombshell, and now he wants to see what I do with it. By his intense uneasy glare, I am guessing that in his mind this blood means cancer. For me, unexpected blood from any orifice – bowels, urine, vagina – might be cancer, and I certainly need to rule it out. But it usually isn't.

'OK. Well, I see a lot of this – there's no need to feel embarrassed at all. And when you say it happens when you go to the loo, do you mean opening your bowels, or peeing?'

'Yes, it's when I open my bowels.' He inhales deeply and slowly through tensed lips, trying to bring his breathing back into line.

This poor man is so nervy that my default GP approach of asking open-ended questions and letting him tell his story doesn't seem likely to be a winner here. Our conversation is too staccato. I think he wants me to take over. Luckily, when someone mentions passing blood from the back passage, every doctor knows what questions to ask, and what needs doing. I know – and he knows – that I will soon have to put my finger up this man's bottom. But for now, I am more than happy to take the wheel and lead the consultation.

'OK. Just a couple of other questions – is it on the paper, or mixed in with the stools?'

I'm trying to be absolutely clear what his symptoms are. No one says 'stools' in real life – but most people at the doctor's seem to understand what it means, and somehow it feels unprofessional to say 'shit' or 'poo', except perhaps with children, or when I gauge it might get a cheap laugh. It's easy to be talking at cross purposes. As a student, I remember having a long conversation with an elderly lady about problems 'down below' and only discovering after half an hour that her 'down below' (anus) was not the same as the 'down below' I had in mind (vagina). I was playing by the rules of polite English society – picking up on her awkwardness and avoiding the issue. As a doctor, you can't afford to do that. Now, with NB, I need to know whether this is just some spotting of bright red blood on the paper after wiping (which often comes from a local surface problem around the anus) or, say, darker blood in the toilet or mixed in with the stools (more likely to have come from higher up inside the bowel itself). It's often hard to gauge how much blood there is though – when even a tiny drop of blood spreads through the water, it can look as if something has just been brutally savaged by a toilet shark.

Passing blood from the back passage (rectal bleeding) is one of our 'red flags'. Red flags, or 'alarm symptoms', are the symptoms or signs that should put every doctor on high alert for a potentially serious problem, particularly cancer. Other red flags when someone has bowel symptoms are unexplained weight loss, or loss of appetite (both can be signs of cancer). Some will seem like red flags to patients too, and trigger a visit to the doctor – but others often won't, for example a change of bowel habit – particularly towards looser or more frequent stools for more than four weeks. When a patient mentions a red-flag symptom my ears prick up. It'll usually mean checking for other red flags, a thorough examination and probably investigations. On the one hand, red flags make me anxious and concerned for the patient about what they might herald; on the other, like a pilot in an emergency, it now becomes very clear what I need to do. It's the GP equivalent of fly-by-wire. The trick is being alarmed enough to be alert, but not so worried that I lose professional focus.

My job as a generalist can seem a bit like finding needles in haystacks. Red flags can help me find them. For example, each of the 43,000 general practitioners in the UK will see about seven new cancers, three to four strokes, and five to six heart attacks each year, assuming he or she is looking after an average of 2000 patients. But the vast majority of patients I see will not have a serious life-threatening disease. The average full-time GP in the UK will see just one new case of bowel cancer each year – but many more people with rectal bleeding from other causes. So the bulk of people with bleeding from the back passage will not have cancer; most bleeding from the back passage is caused by non-cancerous conditions like piles (haemorrhoids), anal fissures (tears), inflammatory bowel disease (inflammation of the bowel, including colitis and Crohn's disease), benign polyps (small growths), or diverticular disease (pouches coming off the bowel wall). Surveys suggest that most people with rectal bleeding won't even bother to see their doctor about it.

Fortunately there are researchers in primary care who specialise in working out how reliable red-flag signs are in predicting serious disease. They analyse symptoms from the records of thousands of patients and come up with a measure called the positive predictive value. This is the proportion of those with the symptom (rectal bleeding) who actually have the disease (in this case bowel cancer). In a recent review of studies looking at this, researchers have estimated that in general practice, bleeding from the back passage has a positive predictive value of up to 5 per cent. So, overall, out of a hundred patients coming to see the GP with rectal bleeding, up to five will have bowel cancer. The risk increases with age, both in men and women. Other red-flag symptoms for bowel problems are less valuable as predictors of cancer: abdominal pain alone, for example, has a positive predictive value of up to 2 per cent, and weight loss is up to 3 per cent. But anaemia seems to have a positive predictive value of up to 5.8 per cent, again increasing with age. And if you combine red-flag symptoms – for example weight loss as well as rectal bleeding – the risk of cancer increases. Through this sort of research we're slowly building a more accurate picture of how good all these red-flag symptoms are at predicting serious disease. What used to be an educated hunch for the 1950s GP is now a rather more robust estimate. Many of our modern clinical guidelines – including those for suspected colorectal cancer – are based on these measurements. The threshold for urgent referral to a specialist is getting lower too – the latest NICE (The National Institute for Health and Care Excellence) guidelines now recommend referral at a 3 per cent risk of cancer, which means that only around one in thirty-three patients with symptoms that may be caused by cancer and who we refer for specialist assessment will actually have cancer. So Mr NB is right to come and get this checked out, and I need to assess his symptoms thoroughly. But from my standpoint, it's still much more likely that this isn't cancer.

I run through my red-flag questions.

'Can I just ask some specific questions about your bowels?'

'Yes, sure.'

'Have you noticed any change in your bowel habit – perhaps going more often than usual, or looser than usual, or perhaps more constipated?'

I always feel the need to spell those subtleties out. I suspect lots of people would think a change in bowel habit would only refer to how frequently they go. NB says he has perhaps been a tiny bit constipated on one or two occasions recently – but still opening his bowels the normal amount for him, once a day. (People sometimes think that there is a fixed definition of a normal bowel habit – once a day for example. That might be normal for some people, but bowel habits vary from person to person. For some people normal means opening their bowels several times a day, for others maybe once every other day. What's more important is that your bowel habits are following a regular pattern and that there's not been any significant change from what's normal for you.)

No major change, NB reports. All other relevant red flags are negative. He hasn't had any pain (occasionally cancers, and some forms of inflammatory bowel disease such as Crohn's or Ulcerative Colitis, can cause pain and bleeding, as can diverticulitis, inflammation of small 'diverticula', or pouches, coming off the bowel wall).

I am now feeling NB's tension mounting – his eyes seem to get wider with every question I ask. The loudest messages are often the unspoken ones. I've probably done too much quick-fire questioning; I need to find out what's on his mind. I failed to react to his earlier cue – the nervous breathing. I could have picked up on it then, but I got side-tracked by the medical details. Now I've got the picture, I can go back and ask what's bothering him.

'When you get blood on the paper, it's quite alarming, isn't it? Lots of people I see are worried it might be something serious.'

'Well, yes, of course. Obviously you worry about that.'

'Was there anything particular on your mind – it just helps me to know.'

'Well, obviously you worry about cancer and things. My father died of cancer.'

I know some patients think these are stupid questions. The 'obviously' says it all. But I also know from experience that not everyone holds the same concerns about the same symptoms. I am constantly amazed by what people think might be causing their symptoms, or how some people are completely unsuspecting about the most alarming signs. For example, a paralysis of one side of the body – put down to a minor arm injury. Or severe long-standing cardiac chest pain attributed to indigestion. I've heard of widespread, even ulcerating, cancers described as 'sores'. So I don't take anything for granted any more. I ask with a genuinely open mind, at the risk of sounding dim or patronising.

For some patients, just saying the word 'cancer' out loud, or sharing worries that have been bottled up for months, can be a huge relief. Worries have a habit of growing out of proportion, particularly when they are allowed to fester unchallenged inside your mind. Some people are visibly shaking with fear as they tell me about their symptoms. In NB's case, it's great to see the relief on his face when he finally spits out his story. And it certainly helps me to know about his dad, and his worries about cancer.

(*three minutes*)

We spend a little while exploring his father's cancer – kidney, not bowel – and I explain that I will ask him some questions and examine him carefully with that in mind – though I think it's very unlikely that cancer is the cause. He seems to have relaxed a little since we have got our cards on the table.

I need to know whether he has any other 'local' symptoms; in other words, symptoms limited to a particular part of the body. In this case, it would help me to know if he has any itching or soreness around the anus. Haemorrhoids, or 'piles', can cause itching or soreness, along with occasional bleeding. They're probably the commonest cause of rectal bleeding I see. Piles are swellings that contain enlarged blood vessels, found inside the rectum or around the anus. You could think of them as varicose veins of the anus. Another common cause is an anal fissure – a small tear in the anus – which can be extremely painful, particularly after opening the bowels. They are often caused by constipation and they usually heal after a week or two. He says he is a bit sore and occasionally itchy around his bottom. In someone his age, small amounts of bright red rectal bleeding with local anal symptoms points much more towards piles or a fissure than something like cancer. I am veering towards piles. I'll examine him with piles in mind – but with nothing ruled out yet.

'OK, so I'd like to examine you, if that's all right? Now this will mean putting a gloved finger in your bottom.'

He shuffles uncomfortably in his plastic NHS chair.

'Yes, I thought you'd have to do that.'

'Have you had this done before?'

'No. First time.' He looks like he might be sick.

'It shouldn't be painful. A little uncomfortable maybe. But it'll only take a few seconds and then it'll all be over. OK?'

'I don't envy you doing that at this time in the morning!'

Quite a few people say they feel sorry for me having to examine them in this way, especially so early in the morning. I tell them not to apologise; it's what we are trained for and I do many such examinations each week. It's not my favourite pastime, admittedly, but it becomes a bit like changing your own child's nappy – part of the accepted routine. I adopt a detached professionalism. I feel much sorrier for him. I know people worry about passing wind – or worse – when they are being examined. Yes, it sometimes happens (it's fairly run of the mill during childbirth too), and I know that feeling of slight bowel insecurity, having had the examination myself. So I sometimes mention that that's normal and not to worry about it. And since a colleague told me how one patient asked him, during the procedure, whether he had a glove on, I now always say that I will insert a 'gloved' finger.

'Oh it's all routine for me – just part of the job. Now, I'm supposed to ask if you would like a chaperone to be in the room, or are you OK to carry on?'

'Oh, no. That's fine.'

We now have very clear guidance on using chaperones (impartial observers) for all intimate examinations. When I was a trainee we wouldn't use chaperones as routine – only when we judged the situation to be potentially awkward or risky. I guess we were more cavalier back then. But things changed in the UK following an independent inquiry into the conduct of Clifford Ayling, a general practitioner from Kent. In 2000 Dr Ayling was convicted of thirteen counts of indecent assault on female patients in his care, was sent to prison for four years, and struck off the medical register. Following a public inquiry in 2004 into his misconduct, the Ayling Report made several recommendations to try to avoid similar situations happening again, including how and when chaperones should be used. Now I am supposed to offer all patients – male or female, and whether the same gender as the doctor or not – a chaperone for examinations of intimate parts such as breast, rectum or genitals. This is mainly to reassure patients, to respect their dignity, and attend to their comfort. But having an impartial observer is also for my benefit – to discourage false accusations or complaints. In reality, though, it can be awkward asking someone if they would like a chaperone. Somehow it implies a lack of trust. Many patients reject the offer anyway – they find having an observer in the room intrusive and embarrassing. In that case I still have to record in the notes that I offered one, and that the patient declined. I am quite happy to proceed with this examination without one though – the patient is a man, about my age, who understands what's going to happen and why, has given consent and just wants to get on with it. I'm trusting my instincts. In any case, when people do request a chaperone, it often means a delay – trained chaperones aren't always available at the drop of a hat – so with time ticking by, I am OK with skipping it.

(*five minutes*)

Since medical school I have had it drummed into me that an abdominal examination is not complete without putting a finger into the back passage. If I don't do this, I could miss vital clues – from suspicious lumps or an enlarged prostate to simple haemorrhoids. As our tutors used to say: 'Put your finger in it – or you'll put your foot in it!'

I must have done many hundreds of digital rectal examinations (digital referring to the finger, nothing electronic). I am totally focused on inspecting and then feeling the rectum, ticking off a mental checklist as I go. I cannot afford to miss anything. The same is true for a breast or genital examination. And when you've had to empty someone's bowels by hand, remove shards of glass from a woman's vagina, or drain a large breast abscess, there really is little that will shock you.

'Right, pop up on the couch here.' I don't know why I say 'pop up'; I guess I'm trying to sound friendly and unthreatening.

'If you could lie on your side, facing the window, that would be great. You don't have to take anything off – just drop your trousers and pants to below your knees. Then what really helps me is if you pull your knees right up to your chest. So you're in a sort of foetal position, like this.'

I mime the position alongside the couch, close the clinical curtain, and prepare my gloves and gel. Perhaps it's because people have seen it on US television programmes and they are distracted, but, despite my instructions, quite a few patients still lie face down with their bottom sticking in the air, or they stand up, hands on the couch and legs apart, as if they are about to be frisked at the roadside by the California Highway Patrol. I have done this spiel so many times; I have to be careful not to sound blasé. After all, for the patient, it's the first time.

As always, the first step is 'inspection' – just looking. Are there any obvious rashes around the anus? Any peri-anal warts ('peri' just means 'around' – so warts around the anus)? Any fissures (tears), or external haemorrhoids (piles)? Nothing obvious.

'OK. I'm putting some gel on the glove and gently putting it inside the back passage now. Let me know if it's painful, and I'll stop.'

I wait for the circular sphincter muscle to relax a little, and then I'm in. (I know this will sound weird, but the anal sphincter really is an astonishingly impressive design. Even the brightest medical engineering minds haven't managed to create a bionic version that works quite as well. A muscular ring which holds everything in, water-tight, until the precise moment you want to let something out. It's something you just take for granted until it's damaged in some way – perhaps from childbirth, nerve damage or complications from a bowel operation.)

I am now feeling, systematically, for any lumps in the lower part of the bowel (rectum). The walls of the rectum should be smooth. If there was a tumour, it would stand proud from the bowel wall and might feel ragged or rough. I imagine a clock and make sure I sweep past 12 o'clock, 3, 6 and 9, all as far as my finger will go. For most people that's about 8–9 cm. My index finger is quite long – around 10.5 cm (I remember being labelled an 'outlier' in a biology experiment at school – my finger length being outside of the normal range). But here's the problem with rectal examinations as a test for bowel cancer: they are only as good as the length of your finger. Even with my ten-centimetre digit, I can never feel more than a tiny percentage of the colon (the colon is about one and a half metres long). I have heard of doctors feeling nothing suspicious when they inserted their finger, but then a subsequent, more thorough, examination at the hospital with a colonoscopy (a tiny camera on the end of a long flexible telescope) finding a tumour at 11 or 12 cm – just out of reach of their fingertip. That doesn't make a digital rectal examination worthless, but you can see why a normal finding can only reassure me – and you – about bowel cancers to a certain extent.

Because NB is a man, I also feel for his prostate gland. That's prostate, not prostrate with an 'r', as many patients seem to call it. Though, on reflection, for most men who come to see me, prostate and prostrate mean roughly the same thing; lying down in a position of submission. I'm feeling the gland through the front wall of his lower bowel. It's on the side facing his tummy. The gland is about the size of a walnut in its shell – I can feel about two to four centimetres of it usually, and it should be smooth and rubbery, a bit like the tip of your nose. As I push my finger in up to the webbing, I am mentally visualising the gland. I have seen loads of real prostate glands during operations and when I dissected a dead body as a medical student. We also sat for hours in a pathology museum at medical school, surrounded by bottled specimens floating in formaldehyde. I've seen many illustrations in textbooks and websites, and images of the gland on various scans. So I suppose I am comparing the picture my fingertip is creating as it sweeps over the surface of the gland with a composite of all those images. I am feeling for the sulcus – a groove down the middle of the gland. I am checking that the texture is normal – I don't want it to feel extremely hard, and I don't want to feel any craggy bits. Those point to cancer. Though, again, this examination on its own is not reliable enough to pick up all prostate cancers. For a start, I can only feel the edges and back-facing side of the gland. There's about 15 per cent of the gland that you just can't feel with a finger. Early prostate cancers aren't possible to feel either – by the time I can feel any changes, the cancer is likely to be fairly advanced. Even in the hands of expert urologists, studies have shown that they often can't even agree on what they can feel.

What I am more likely to detect, especially in older men, is a straightforward enlarged prostate. It gets bigger as men get older, and sometimes that can cause problematic urinary symptoms because the urinary pipe flows right through the middle of the prostate. It's a bit like a pipe going through the centre of a big inflatable rubber ring; as the ring gets increasingly pumped up, the pipe in the middle gets squeezed. Experienced urologists like to estimate the volume of the gland by a digital rectal examination – they write in their letters 'the prostate has a volume of X mls', as if it had been measured with a computer-guided laser.

Teaching today's medical students the art and science of the digital rectal exam is a challenge. They desperately need to practise but, naturally, not every patient is keen to be the one they practise on. Nor can I tell, as their teacher, whether a student is doing it right – I can't see what they are feeling, or which bits they are probing with their fingertip. When I was training thirty years ago, and sadly more recently than that, students were sometimes invited by their consultant to practise intimate examinations on patients while they were under anaesthetic for an operation, without the patient's explicit consent. Even if you accept that ethical values change over the years, that was a breach of the trust and respect that underpins the doctor–patient relationship. It certainly shouldn't happen without consent nowadays. Modern medical schools today have plastic models of bottoms with various-sized prostate glands to feel – but they aren't hugely realistic. They'd just about do for a stag-night comedy costume. And, importantly, these don't teach doctors how to communicate with the human attached to the bottom. Researchers at my institution, Imperial College in London, are developing a more realistic training model using computer modelling and haptic technology, which simulates touch and feel, like an advanced computer game. Students put their finger in a special port, and what they feel is based on detailed computer models of real prostates of various sorts. It's early days, but this sort of high-fidelity simulation could make life easier for students – and patients of course – in the future.

I snap off my gloves so they are inside out and dump them in the clinical bin. I wash my hands, with soap then sanitiser gel. I have a quick feel of his abdomen, checking there are no obvious masses, or enlargement of any organs like the liver (top right of the abdomen, tucked under the ribcage).

(*seven minutes*)

'Have a seat. So, I'm pleased to say that was all normal – nothing nasty to feel, no obvious sinister lumps, and no skin tears for example.'

'Oh, good.' The visible loosening of tension in his body tells me he's more relieved than he sounds.

'So, look. There's nothing here to suggest bowel cancer – which obviously you were concerned about. You don't have the typical warning symptoms like a significant change in bowel habit, or weight loss, and you've only noticed blood a couple of times over two weeks. Everything was normal when I examined you. So I think your soreness, itching and slight constipation probably all point to haemorrhoids – piles. That's much more the picture here. I wouldn't necessarily expect to feel internal piles on examination. Do you know much about piles?'

We are taught that the first step in giving information to patients is finding out what they already know. It's tempting to dump on him everything I know about piles, but I really need to start in receiver rather than transmit mode. He says he doesn't know much, so we have a piles talk. 'Try to avoid constipation by increasing your fluid intake, and increase the fibre in your diet.' He thinks he could do that. He should try to avoid 'straining at stool' – sitting and straining for ages on the toilet, with or without reading material. He's not so sure about that one. He can use laxatives if needed, but they're often not required. I give him some suppositories with local anaesthetic and a steroid in them, which can ease discomfort and itching and reduce the swelling. I offer him a leaflet – we know that patients only remember about 10 per cent of what we say, particularly when they are anxious.

If he asked me whether I could guarantee, 100 per cent, that he didn't have bowel cancer, I would have to say no. They say general practice is the art of managing uncertainty, and it often feels like that. Without sending everyone with minor bowel symptoms for a colonoscopy – an unpleasant, costly, invasive procedure with its own risks – the patient and I have to live with the very small risk that he may have cancer. In a system with a limited budget, testing people with extremely low risk of cancer would mean that people at high risk would have to wait much longer. Even if we tested everyone who has rectal bleeding with a colonoscopy, we'd miss some cancers, including those that don't reveal themselves with bleeding. Some people would even come to harm, unnecessarily. But with a detailed history, scanning for red flags, and a careful examination, the idea is that the risk is so vanishingly small that it's a risk we can all live with. Throughout the consultation, I am assessing that risk – not by working out the odds myself, but by drawing on a range of skills and guidelines based on those statistics.

For suspected bowel cancer, for example, we have a strict set of criteria by which to judge whether someone should be sent for urgent investigation (within two weeks). They are pretty detailed, and your GP should know them or be able to refer to them quickly. For instance, at the moment in the NHS, for someone under fifty to qualify for the suspected bowel cancer 'two-week rule', they would need to have rectal bleeding and another red-flag symptom like unexplained abdominal pain, change in bowel habit, weight loss, or anaemia. Anyone forty or over with unexplained weight loss and abdominal pain would qualify. Anyone fifty or over with unexplained rectal bleeding, or someone sixty and over with iron deficiency anaemia, or a change in bowel habit or anyone with a positive test for blood in the faeces would be included. As would anyone at any age with a mass in the rectum or abdomen.

All these criteria are flickering through my mind throughout the consultation. On the basis of his history and my examination, and given NB's age (thirty-six), I am happy to put his symptoms down to haemorrhoids for now. But bearing in mind his cancer worries and the limitations of rectal examination, I will make a routine referral to the bowel specialists to make a more formal diagnosis. Guidelines are only guidelines after all.

Overall, cancer survival in the UK has doubled in the last forty years – but not enough to catch up with levels achieved in many European countries a decade earlier. In the UK, five-year survival rates from colon cancer is lower than in many countries of similar wealth, and that's partly down to delayed diagnosis. For example, survival from colon cancer at five years in the UK was recently estimated at 54 per cent (cancer patients do not all die from their cancer and that figure takes account of death from other causes). But Sweden, Norway, the Netherlands, France, Finland and Italy were all doing better than that a decade earlier. Now Italy, Finland and Sweden all have five-year survival rates of 63 per cent, and it's 60 per cent in France and the Netherlands. In the United States, the figure is nearer 65 per cent. With our two-week rapid referrals for suspected cancers, and our guidelines on who to refer urgently, things are improving. But the guidelines only really help with the more typical presentations, and there's still much work to be done. As a nation we probably don't always go to the doctor soon enough with symptons that could represent early cancer.

I try to tame some of this uncertainty I'm feeling by safety-netting.

'If your symptoms haven't settled over the next couple of weeks, or if you develop any other changes in your bowels, please come back and let me know, will you? Or another option would be to refer you to the bowel specialists so they can do a more thorough check, say with a small scope, than I can do in the surgery today. What do you think?'

'Yes, thanks. I think that's probably sensible. Let's do that.'

(***ten minutes***)

Now we're in extra time. I really don't want to start the morning running behind. But the digital gate-crasher on my desk is pestering me to check his blood pressure and cholesterol. I can do these pretty quickly. I wouldn't suggest them if the bowel diagnosis had been more serious – it would have seemed callous. But NB is in a pretty good mood now, and after a finger up the bottom and cancer anxiety, a blood pressure cuff should be a breeze.

'Do you mind if I measure your blood pressure? The computer's reminding me that we haven't checked it for quite a while.'

'No, go ahead.' He seems pleased with my thoroughness.

Luckily it's fine. Well, pretty much fine: 140/87 – we'd like it lower but that will do (below 140/90 is OK for most people). We order a cholesterol blood test for later too.

While I'm taking his blood pressure, he says, 'Oh, by the way, one of your colleagues said they would refer me to the hospital to remove a fatty lump on my back – that was a few weeks ago – but I haven't heard anything yet. Wondered if you could chase that up for me?'

It feels like I'm getting several requests a day to chase up referrals that have vanished into the great NHS black hole. I write it down as another task in my red book. 'Chase up referral for lipoma.' What a waste of everyone's time.

After he's gone, I write up the notes. Two entries – one about the rectal bleeding, and one about the blood pressure and cholesterol. This makes it easier to make sense of later; and makes sure the practice gets the payments it is due for looking after his blood pressure and cardio-vascular risk.

I haven't done anything heroic in the last thirteen minutes. This time, like most of the time, I didn't spot a cancer. I didn't make a fancy diagnosis and I didn't perform a clever procedure. Instead I've listened, hopefully asked the right questions, and stuck an educated finger up NB's bottom. The real kick for me is using those skills to take the sting out of someone's worry. NB is visibly happier. And I've made sure he's not running a dangerously high blood pressure or cholesterol level – not glamorous, but potentially life-saving. I hope I've calmed things down, ruled things out, prevented trouble ahead. If I have, it was time well spent. *If* I have . . .

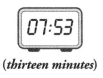

(*thirteen minutes*)

Chapter 3

Ms AF

(running four minutes late)

Doctor view

Appointment time: 7:50
Name: Ms AF
Age: 29 years old
Occupation: Media producer
Past medical history:
  Irritable bowel syndrome
  Appendicectomy (age 14)
Medication:
  No regular medication
Reminders:
  None
Last consultation:
  Nine months ago, for repeat prescription
  of the oral contraceptive pill.

Patient view

Ms AF has had a sore throat for twelve hours. It's not getting better, and she has an important job interview in three days' time. She just wants some strong antibiotics like she had last year – they did the trick within a day. She's tried all the usual over-the-counter remedies but they only work for a very short time, and she really needs this to be better soon. She is in a bit of a hurry as she has an important meeting to go to.

Ms AF has straw-coloured hair in a neat bob, and she's wearing a smart dark blue work dress. I call her name and she's off the waiting-room bench like a dog out of the traps. I have to accelerate, like an Olympic speed walker, to make it back to my consulting room before she does. I win – just – and as I am gesturing to her to sit down, she starts . . .

'I've got a terrible sore throat and absolutely *nothing* is working. It's just getting worse. So I really need you to give me something stronger.'

Part of me breathes a sigh of relief when the problem is a sore throat. It's not glamorous *House*-style medicine, but I can usually catch up on time and I don't have to think too hard. I imagine it's the equivalent of a blocked sink for a plumber, or a faulty spark plug for a mechanic. But I bet even blocked sinks and faulty spark plugs can be more or less challenging, depending on who they belong to – and it's the same with sore throats.

When I see a patient with a sore throat, I become very focused on finding out early on what they are expecting from their ten minutes. You might think that once you've seen one sore throat you've seen them all, but patients have all sorts of different agendas. Here are just a few I've encountered: 'I just want to check that it doesn't need anti-biotics'; 'I need it better by Friday for a job interview'; 'I need antibiotics because it was the only thing that worked last time'; 'I think I am getting too many sore throats and my immune system is weak'; 'I need a tonsillectomy'; 'I think it could be glandular fever.' My agenda is: I need to know early on which road we are likely to travel down in the next ten minutes; they are often very different journeys.

AF has dropped a heavy hint that she wants something stronger – usually that means antibiotics. At least she hasn't beaten around the bush. But her forthright style is making me bristle. I think it's the phrase 'I really need you to . . .' which has pushed my buttons. I'm proud to be a public servant, but not in the slave sense. Her words make me feel like her minion. I have to consciously maintain a profes-sional approach. For me, the best way (and I recommend this to medi-cal students and trainees) is to think like Columbo – the American TV detective – and become curious about her behaviour rather than getting caught up in it. It's a kind of detached concern, a focus on

47

clues. The first step is to recognise how I'm feeling, what my internal weather pattern is like. Then I start wondering why she's coming over so pushy to me, why she wants something stronger, and why she might think antibiotics are the answer. She becomes more of a puzzle than an annoyance.

'OK, and when you say "something stronger", did you have something in mind?'

'Well, I really need antibiotics. I've had exactly the same symptoms before and it was only strong antibiotics that got rid of it.'

'Was that from us?'

'Yes, it was last year.'

'OK. Let me have a look.'

A year ago we gave her phenoxymethylpenicillin 500 mg four times a day for ten days – which is fairly standard antibiotic treatment for tonsillitis. The notes – from a colleague – describe the typical signs of classic tonsillitis with swollen tonsils, a fever, and exudate on the tonsils (white patches or spots). She'd had her symptoms for five days before getting antibiotics last time. When she came after two days, we didn't give her any. Maybe that's behind her brusqueness today. The question now is whether she has classic tonsillitis needing antibiotics again, or whether this time it's more likely to be a virus which should sort itself out without resorting to unnecessary medication. And if it does look like a virus, how am I going to persuade her that she really doesn't need antibiotics?

Gathering information about a sore throat is straightforward enough – I take a history and examine the patient, looking for specific signs such as fever, glands in the neck, and exudate on the tonsils. My questions are designed to find out how the problem is affecting her everyday life (including at work), whether she has any associated symptoms such as a cough, and whether she has a temperature. With that information, I can refer to clear evidence-based guidelines called the Centor criteria (after the researcher who originally described them) on which sore throats are likely to benefit from antibiotics, and which simply need the usual advice about symptom relief, like painkillers (some people find gargling with salt water or mouthwashes or sucking throat lozenges helpful, but there is little robust evidence that it makes much difference) for example. I don't literally refer to these guidelines – they lurk in my psyche as a mental checklist.

The Centor criteria were developed to predict the chances of a sore throat being caused by a streptococcal bacterial infection, rather than something else – usually a virus. There are four criteria: the presence of tonsillar exudate; the presence of tender (sore to the touch) lymph nodes in the front part of the neck; a history of fever; and the absence of a cough. Tender lymph nodes and fever are usually a sign that the body is fighting off infection, and if you have a cough alongside your sore throat the chances are greater that it's all caused by a virus (viruses rarely attack just one bit of the body – if they were bombs, they'd be more like carpet bombs than laser-guided missiles). If you meet three or four of these Centor criteria then there is a good chance (40–60 per cent) that you may have an infection caused by a common sore throat bacterium (called group A beta-haemolytic streptococcus). If you only meet one or two of the criteria, then there's an 80 per cent chance that you don't have this bug, and therefore that antibiotics are unlikely to be helpful. It's not foolproof, but it does give me some guidance, based on evidence, when it comes to deciding who will benefit from antibiotics and who probably won't. That's important, because by prescribing unnecessary antibiotics I encourage the development of bacteria that are resistant to our usual antibiotics. It's a massive and growing problem.

The Centor criteria are an example of a clinical prediction rule – a formal type of pattern recognition based on a well-defined and widely tested series of similar cases. When it comes to clinical prediction rules for sore throats, there's a new kid on the block; recent research suggests that one called the Fever Pain clinical score might be more accurate than the Centor criteria.

GPs use lots of different clinical prediction rules for all sorts of different situations. For example, the Ottawa ankle rules to predict whether someone has broken their ankle rather than sprained it; the ABCD score for assessing someone's risk of having a stroke; or the Wells score for helping decide whether someone might have a deep vein thrombosis in their leg. They can be a great help and comfort when I'm deciding such things as whether to send someone to hospital or back home, but as more and more spring up we need to know which ones are most useful and how best to use them in practice.

AF tells me she doesn't think she's had a fever, and she hasn't had a cough. The sore throat came on only twelve hours ago. Just from her story so far, she doesn't look like she'll be hitting the Centor jackpot.

(*three minutes*)

I save my throat examination till last – for me that's the big 'reveal', like the final scene of a murder mystery. I gather clues from a patient's story, and other bits of the examination first. I suppose it keeps me entertained, and it's a bit of a test of my clinical acumen – can I work out what someone's tonsils will look like before I shine my torch on them? So I talk AF through my examination, simultaneously checking for her consent.

'Can I just feel for any lymph glands in your neck?'

Lymph glands and lymph are a major part of the body's immune system. There are clusters of lymph nodes in the neck, as well as in the groin and the armpits. Normally they are about pea-size, and occasionally you can feel them. But when you have a throat infection, the nearby glands swell up as they swing into action, producing white cells and antibodies to fight off any local attack. They can get as big as a marble and can be quite sore. Usually they shrink back down to their normal size within a week or so of an infection. There are other more serious but much less common causes of swollen lymph glands – like cancers, lymphomas and leukaemias. A general virus such as flu or glandular fever can cause the lymph glands all over your body to swell up. Right now though, I am using the neck glands as a marker of local infection – another clue as to what is going on.

I have been taught a systematic way to explore a patient's neck lymph nodes, checking each cluster or chain of nodes in turn. Some are best felt from behind the patient as they are seated, but I need to warn AF what I'm doing because it could seem as though I am about to strangle her. The tips of my fingers gently probe the area, marking out the edges of any nodes, checking how large they are, how firm or soft, and noting whether they are tender for the patient. Having felt thousands of necks in this way, and casting my mind back to deadly anatomy sessions with corpses, I know roughly where the main clusters are, what 'normal' feels like, and which areas of the head and neck they serve (for example, enlarged nodes at the back of the head often suggest a scalp infection). Her anterior cervical nodes (the ones at the front of her neck) are slightly swollen and a little tender.

I check her temperature using an electronic infrared thermometer in her ear. Normal range.

Now time to open up the bonnet and take a look. (I am guessing that without a fever, without feeling generally unwell, with only a twelve-hour history, and with fairly unimpressive lymph nodes, AF won't have the swollen, inflamed tonsils and exudate of acute bacterial tonsillitis. I'd bet at least a fiver on it.)

'Say "Air".'

Asking patients to say 'Ahh' makes me feel like a real doctor, and patients are expecting it. But I have discovered that by saying 'Air', I get a much better view of someone's tonsils on both sides. Saying 'air' with your mouth wide open lifts the soft palate up, revealing more of the tonsils. I try not to use a tongue depressor – the wooden lollipop stick that presses your tongue out of the way – I hated it when I was a child because it made me gag. But sometimes I do need to use one in order to see things properly. I warn people they may gag – and that's normal. It's an automatic reflex. In fact sometimes we test for it deliberately to check the nerve supply is working properly. In the UK in general practice we don't usually take throat swabs any more (an elongated cotton bud, used to take bacterial samples from the surface of the tonsils) – the results take several days to come back and rarely alter our management. They can't distinguish between a streptococcal infection and people who just carry the bug in their throat without it causing infection (between 6 and 40 per cent of us carry the bug without problems – 'asymptomatic carriers'). I sometimes do a throat swab in tricky cases, if the patient is very ill or if they haven't responded as expected to antibiotics. In the United States, doctors often use rapid antigen tests – a throat swab that can give results in a matter of minutes. They may be helpful but recent research shows no clear benefit over using a clinical score alone.

I can see AF's tonsils, two pitted fleshy lumps of meat on either side of the back of the throat. Her uvula, like a soft pink punch-bag, dangles down, right in the middle between them. Her tonsils look a brighter red than normal – perhaps mildly inflamed, at worst. No exudate though. Centor score 2.

(*five minutes*)

Whenever I look at tonsils, I am glad that part of my GP training included three months as a junior hospital doctor in Ear, Nose and Throat surgery (or Otolaryngology, to give it its formal name). I came to know the tonsil intimately – in all its guises. I remember terrifying nights hovering over the telephone wondering if I should call the consultant, looking after children who had had their tonsils removed during the day – watching for life-threatening bleeding (as opposed to the normal bleeding you'd expect after having glands spooned out of the back of your throat).

I did once have to call the consultant in at night so we could take a child back to theatre for an emergency operation to stop the bleeding. Then there were the children with unfeasibly large tonsils that touched in the middle and interfered with their breathing – anything that compromises the airway is scary for the doctor as well as the patient. It was for me, anyway. Often they don't need removing, but very occasionally they do become an emergency. And the worst, for me, was an abscess on the tonsil (a quinsy), a rare but serious complication of tonsillitis. Patients are frequently in extreme pain from a build-up of pus around the tonsil. When you look inside the mouth, the tonsil is extremely swollen and the uvula is often swollen and pushed over to one side. My job was to drain the abscess by inserting a scalpel into it. We used only a local anaesthetic spray. I had to pierce exactly the right spot, and I'd taped up the scalpel so that only the tip was exposed – this was to make sure it didn't go in too deeply and puncture an artery. My heart was pounding; the patient was in agony. But get this procedure right, and, apart from the foul taste of pus and blood once it is incised, it's the most dramatic instant relief for the patient that I have seen.

I don't drain tonsillar abscesses in general practice – but the experience has given me the confidence to diagnose a few, and puts twelve-hour 'sore throats' into perspective. One of the endless fascinations of general practice is why some patients seem to come in with 'trivia' while others stoically sit at home with chest pains, determined not to bother the doctor. This first hit home for me when, as a hospital doctor, I was caring for two patients in adjacent cubicles. One, a young woman, was whining loudly about a barely visible rash she'd had for a few days; the other, a factory worker, thought I was overreacting when I suggested we should try to sew back his fingers, which had been severed by a packaging machine. I felt they could both do with being introduced to each other.

But when I see someone in the practice who might strike some people as being a bit pathetic – or even breathtakingly feeble – I draw on some of the medical sociology we get taught in our training. We know that in the UK, for example, only a tiny proportion of people with a cough will go to see their doctor – as GPs we see only the tip of the symptom iceberg. Of the estimated 48 million episodes of a cough each year, 24 million people will self-medicate, and only about 12 million will end up making an appointment with the doctor.

There are lots of different theories and models that attempt to explain why some people go to the doctor and others don't. One is the idea of a lay referral system – a network of family members and authoritative lay people who patients 'consult' before seeing the doctor. How many of these lay contacts they make before seeing their GP depends on how similar the social background is between the patient and the doctor; people from higher socioeconomic backgrounds seem to need less 'permission' from others to attend. It's also noticeable that family members tend to behave in similar ways when it comes to their health – perhaps steered by a common, inherited, in-house lay referral system.

Then there are 'Zola's triggers'. In an influential research paper in 1973, Zola made the point that symptoms alone were not enough to make someone decide to see the doctor – there were other key triggers at play. He identified five types of trigger: an interpersonal crisis (for example, a death in the family); interference with social or personal relations ('I can't look after the kids any more'); sanctioning (pressure or advice from others to attend – 'the wife told me to come', or 'you look awful, have you seen a doctor?'); interference with vocational or physical activity ('I can't do my normal exercise any more'); and what he called temporalising – the setting of a deadline ('if it's not better by Monday, I'll see the doctor'). His point, radical at the time, was that most people make rational decisions to seek (or delay seeking) medical help – at least in terms of their own beliefs and values.

In today's ethically diverse society, different cultural beliefs or norms can also explain differences in patients' health behaviours. One study, for example, found that British Bangladeshis with diabetes had a range of folk health beliefs – some felt that their lack of sweating in the British cold weather was bad for their metabolism and that if they could only return to warmer climates they would be cured. Many countries don't have a GP-based health system – we can often find ourselves explaining the role of the British GP. No, you don't have to pay. No, you don't need to go straight to a paediatrician about your child, or a gynaecologist for your smear test.

The bottom line here for me is that, whatever I may feel inside, it really isn't helpful to be too judgemental about patients who seem to come for the slightest thing – or never come until it's too late. There are so many influences at play, and I see my job as trying to understand what they are so I can help the patient as much as I can. Sometimes that does mean explaining what is appropriate use of a health system that's free at the point of care – but often it is more about understanding and firm, clear reassurance.

Now I want to get underneath AF's hurry and need. It's ICE time: I need to unearth her Ideas, Concerns and Expectations. I must choose my words carefully though, to avoid irritating her – on the other hand,

I am the guardian of a precious and powerful resource. I would be compromising my professional integrity and duty if I were to hand out antibiotics like sweeties. Like using a sledgehammer to crack a nut. And I'd be contributing to that growing problem of resistant bacteria as well as risking possible side effects, such as diarrhoea, nausea and rashes. It's in moments like these that I feel the media shouting at me with a megaphone from the sidelines: irresponsible GPs are over-prescribing antibiotics and risking the development of antibiotic resistance. It's no longer a prediction – it's happening now. The world is heading towards a post-antibiotic era, in which common infections and minor injuries, which have been treatable for decades, can once again kill. But believe me, we are fully aware of the risks. We talk about it endlessly, we research the problem, and practise how to tackle the pressures to prescribe. In the UK, unlike some countries, patients must have their antibiotics prescribed by a doctor rather than simply being able to buy them over the counter at the pharmacy. We are on the frontline of this particular battle.

I accept that as a custodian of our antibiotic armoury, I must shoulder some of the blame for the build-up of antibiotic resistance. But I think patients must take some responsibility here too. Part of the problem is that some patients can become very angry or anxious if they are not given antibiotics, even when their symptoms are clearly caused by a virus. Many simply won't accept that viruses get better on their own, and antibiotics don't work for viral infections. They are impatient and want something to get rid of the symptoms NOW. I have resorted to pinning on my wall the average duration of symptoms for the most common viral infections. Somehow it seems to carry more weight if it's printed out, but many people still struggle to believe the figures. You can expect a run-of-the-mill viral cough to last about three weeks. A common cold, about ten to fourteen days. About seven days for your average sore throat.

I often sense confrontation, or even feel its full force. Even a low-grade clash can add many minutes to the appointment and leave me – not to mention the patients in the waiting room – feeling stressed and angry. As a GP, of course I don't want to prescribe antibiotics unnecessarily, but equally I don't want us to fall out and ruin the precious doctor–patient relationship, which could have important implications for the patient's future health. Patients often want something to take away from their visit to the doctor, particularly if they have waited a while to get an appointment. A fascinating study published recently in the *British Journal of General Practice* found that GP practices that prescribe fewer antibiotics tend to get lower patient satisfaction scores; in a sense, we're damned if we do prescribe and damned if we don't. I don't want to get behind schedule either. And there's always a nagging worry that if I refuse to give antibiotics to an insistent patient, sure as hell it'll be that patient who develops complications (which we know are very uncommon) or becomes really unwell.

The uncertainty of medicine, the blame culture and the constant threat of litigation mean that too often my decisions are driven by fear. I've been involved in two or three formal complaints in my career – each one has made me a little more defensive, risk-averse. And as if those experiences were not enough, I hear about fellow doctors being sued, or receive horrific bulletins from medical indemnity organisations, crammed with stories about near misses, injured patients and struck-off doctors. Many doctors are terrified of getting it wrong, getting sued, hitting the headlines, or being investigated by the General Medical Council (GMC). GPs are more likely to be sued than ever before – a full-time GP can expect to receive two clinical negligence claims over a career. Our regulatory bodies are contributing to a climate of fear. A GMC-commissioned review in 2014 found that from 2005 to 2013, twenty-eight doctors died from suicide or suspected suicide while undergoing fitness-to-practise investigations. The majority of doctors who are reported to the GMC are found to have no case to answer. Maybe all this explains why, even though it's not always best for the patient, modern GPs are more likely to play safe, stick to the guidance, refer, prescribe, investigate. In a recent survey, 79 per cent of doctors who had experienced a complaint said they had changed their clinical practice as a result. They used tactics such as avoiding difficult tasks, ordering too many investigations and, in some cases, acting against their professional judgement. In other words: modern defensive medicine. Patients' fears fuel my fears too, and so the cycle continues. I need to learn to live with the uncertainty – and somehow we have to help patients to live with it too.

It's a delicate dance, and often the pragmatic solution is a compromise. Rather than saying an outright 'no' to antibiotics, like a parent to a naughty toddler, I can offer a delayed prescription for antibiotics, only to be used if symptoms are not improving as expected in forty-eight hours or so. This can often defuse a tense stand-off, and the evidence suggests that it cuts antibiotic use, keeps patients satisfied, and doesn't make them any more likely to develop complications from an infection. But, if I'm honest, it's a fudge.

'Now, from what you said earlier, I know you are keen on antibiotics, like you had last time, but fortunately I don't think you will need them this time. I can see that your tonsils are red and swollen – it looks very sore. But you don't have the signs of full-blown tonsillitis caused by bacteria – pus or white spots on the tonsils, fever and so on. Last time you came, you did have those signs – of full-blown tonsillitis – and that is almost certainly why the antibiotics did the trick so quickly. They were treating a bacterial infection. But today it looks as though your sore throat is down to a virus – and of course antibiotics don't have any effect on viruses. So from a clinical standpoint, this should clear up by itself in a few days and we can give you painkillers and so on to help the symptoms – but I don't think antibiotics would do you any good, or make your recovery any quicker.'

'But it's the only thing that works for me,' she snaps back. 'I've got an important job interview in a couple of days and I really need them – I know my body and it's exactly the same as last time. I've tried the ibuprofen and gargling and it just isn't working.'

Here we go. Flak jacket on. I don't relish confrontation – but it looks like we are heading that way. There are occasions when I'd contemplate squaring up to her, but I just don't have time for this right now. Most of my colleagues are tougher than me; a few are more of a pushover. But she is now an informed adult, and, on balance, if she is set on taking antibiotics I am not going to stand in her way. I pick my battles these days – I would draw the line at unnecessary requests for more powerful or potentially addictive medicines like benzodiazepines (tranquillisers such as Diazepam), for example. I give her the delayed script spiel.

When relationships with patients get tricky, we often refer to the work of Eric Berne and his influential book on human relationships called *Games People Play*. Berne, a Canadian psychiatrist, came up with the theory of transactional analysis to explain human behaviour and interactions. It borrows some concepts from the work of Freud. Berne's theory suggests that in any transaction with others, people adopt one of three 'ego-states'. We are either being Parent, Adult or Child. In Parent role, we feel responsible and don't necessarily want to engage in much discussion with our children. We can be strict and controlling. In Child mode we tend to behave, think and feel as we remember childhood to be; sometimes it's the freedom of not having to make important decisions, sometimes the frustration of being told what to do. We can be trusting and accepting – or sulky and irritable. In Adult mode, we make decisions on the basis of rational thought, unclouded by major emotions. We take responsibility for ourselves, we're open to discussion, and we ask for or offer advice or information appropriately. Berne reckons that the roles people play in any situation can either be chosen by ourselves (often unconsciously) or projected onto us by the person we are talking to. We adopt one or other of these states instinctively, based on what we have learned about being a parent, adult or child.

Berne's theory can be very helpful for GPs when consultations don't seem to be working very well. Although we strive for an adult–adult interaction between the doctor and patient, sometimes we find ourselves behaving more like a bossy adult to a child-like patient (even when we don't want to). Or the reverse – we take on the role of a submissive and accepting child when faced with a parent-like patient, telling us what to do. Sometimes Berne's theory can help us analyse the roles we take on during the consultation, and offers ways to encourage a more adult–adult partnership. Why, for example, do some patients act in a very child-like manner? Are they anxious for some reason, perhaps worried about assuming responsibility for their own health? In AF's case, why is she being rather parental? Has she had bad experiences with doctors in the past? Is she frightened of losing control? I might explore that with her next time. How is her behaviour affecting the way I am behaving in this consultation? Do I need to start behaving more like an adult than a child playing to her maternal tune?

'As I have said, I really don't think you need antibiotics this time – you will be able to fight it off on your own. And I don't think they'd make you better any quicker – they may even give you diarrhoea, which I'm afraid would make you worse off for your job interview. But I don't want us to fall out over this. If you are absolutely set on them, could we agree to me giving you a prescription for antibiotics, only to be used if things are not getting better in forty-eight hours or so?'

As I say this, AF's features soften, and I can tell she feels she has got what she wanted. But my professional pride is intact too. It doesn't feel like complete capitulation. I know there's a risk that she might go straight to the pharmacy and cash in her prescription – but the evidence suggests that there's a good chance she won't (fewer than 40 per cent of patients actually use antibiotics when offered a delayed prescription for a cough or sore throat).

(*eight minutes*)

A sore throat – along with other common upper respiratory tract infections (URTIs) such as coughs – is a good example of how, while I sift through the mountains of the mundane, I must always be alert to the life-threatening. Just occasionally – fortunately it is very rare – quite innocuous symptoms like sore throats and coughs will herald a much more serious illness. These days, GPs are taught to pay close attention to the general health of the patient, particularly children who can deteriorate very quickly – heart rate, breathing rate, circulation and oxygen saturation (measured with a tiny digital gadget that clips onto the end of a finger). So if there's any doubt about how sick someone is, I would measure those too. The trouble is, we often see patients early on in an illness, when the cardinal symptoms have not yet developed. No meningitis rash or limb pain, no chickenpox lesions yet, no shingles blisters. That means it's hard to nail the diagnosis, and it's hard to gauge how ill the patient may yet become.

In shadowy corners of my mind are the dark memories of moments when throats haven't behaved as expected. One is a time many years ago when I was at work in an office away from the surgery, and a work friend mentioned that she wasn't feeling great. She said it was a bit like a mini-hangover, and she had a mild sore throat and had lost her voice that morning. With my GP hat on, it sounded to me like a typical viral upper respiratory tract infection; sore throat, headache, a bit fluey, and laryngitis (inflammation of the voice box). Although I couldn't do a proper examination in the office, she didn't seem very sick. I gave her the usual advice to go home and rest; after all, most viral URTIs get better on their own after a few days. She went home, but started vomiting repeatedly. She called her GP, who prescribed an antibiotic – the plan was for her flatmate to collect them from the pharmacist and bring them back with him after work. When he came home he found her barely conscious. The GP made an urgent house call, diagnosed meningitis and called an ambulance. My friend wasn't able to see by this stage. She spent the next week or so in intensive care. Thank God she recovered fully. But I felt awful – for her of course, but also guilty that I hadn't advised her to see a doctor sooner. On reflection, and talking with the doctors who were looking after her in hospital, any self-respecting GP would probably have said the same at that stage of her illness. Even after assessment in the surgery. Sore throat, losing your voice and feeling fluey are common symptoms. They are not common early signs of meningitis, and at that stage of the illness there were few clues as to what was to follow. GPs – and patients – have to live with that kind of uncertainty.

GPs are the risk sink for the health service. That is why we use safety-netting. People joke that GPs say 'take some paracetamol and come back again if doesn't get better'. But this is how we try to grapple with the uncertainty medicine throws up. The skill is in making a safety-net that's fit for purpose and specific – anticipating the worst-case scenarios and spelling them out clearly so the patient understands what to look out for and what to do. In our GP professional exam, the MRCGP (Membership of the Royal College of GPs), which all GPs in the UK are now required to pass before they can practise as a GP, one of the key skills the examiners judge us on is our safety-netting.

'Right now,' I say therefore to AF, 'this looks like a viral sore throat. If I were you, I'd take some simple painkillers like ibuprofen, and use salt water or a simple mouthwash, or lozenges to suck on to relieve the symptoms. But I'd expect it to be getting steadily better over the next three to five days. If that doesn't happen – particularly if you feel unwell in yourself, drowsy, have any trouble with your breathing or swallowing, or start vomiting – then see a doctor straight away. OK?'

'Yes, OK. Thank you.'

'Here's your prescription for antibiotics – only if needed in forty-eight hours or so.' I collect the script from the printer behind me and swivel round triumphantly. This is the traditional full stop in the consultation – the handing over of what she came for. Hopefully it shouts: 'OK, we're done.'

(**ten minutes**)

'Oh yes, while I'm here, I wanted to ask you about something else. I have been trying for a baby for six months now and wanted to get my fertility checked.'

My lips tighten and my smiley goodbye face becomes much more frowny. It's the dreaded 'hand-on-knob' consultation all GPs will recognise. This is when a patient has come with one problem, but then – just as he or she is about to leave – adds another, often bigger, problem (with his or her hand on the door knob, about to leave). It's frequently prefaced with 'while I'm here . . .' – words that nearly always speed up my heart rate.

This can be infuriating for me – it makes me run very late – but I try to bear in mind why patients do this (it's often about gaining trust or courage using a more minor complaint, like a passport, before moving on to something serious). In fact I have used this technique myself, when I was in my teens. I was worried by some tiny white spots on my penis, so plucked up courage to go to see the family GP. But I got the appointment on an asthma ticket – I needed a new inhaler as I'd run out. The GP must have thought 'Oh great, a straightforward asthma review and repeat prescription of an inhaler.' But when all that was done, and I felt comfortable with him, I dropped my penis bombshell, so to speak. It didn't take long actually – they were normal, visible sebaceous glands called Fordyce spots.

The problem with the hand-on-knob consultation is that when you only have ten minutes, you can start running very late if you address the add-on problem properly. Or worse, you try to address it but take potentially risky short-cuts. I find that it's often better to suggest the patient comes back another time so that I can focus fully on the problem, give it the time it deserves.

This time, I decide that we can compromise a little. Fertility consultations are complex and take at least ten minutes. But there are some basic blood tests that usually need doing as routine – sex hormones, thyroid hormones, a full blood count. So I suggest that we can get those done to get the ball rolling, and then she can come back to discuss the results with me another time. I also ask her how long ago she stopped taking the oral contraceptive pill and what is happening to her periods. It's not uncommon for women's periods to stop for several months after coming off the pill – and without periods she is probably not ovulating, which means pregnancy is very unlikely. Her periods are regular though, so we agree to my blood tests and review plan.

All that takes another five minutes. I am now running ten minutes late. I type up her notes furiously, and when I glance at the screen I notice half the entry is in CAPITALS, and I have written 'antibOOtics' and 'exDuate'. Bollocks.

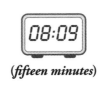

(*fifteen minutes*)

Chapter 4

Mr NA

*(**running ten minutes late**)*

Doctor view

Appointment time: 8.00
Name: Mr NA
Age: 59 years old
Occupation: Business consultant
Past medical history:
Hernia repair
Removal of mole
Fractured fibula
Hay fever
Medication:
No regular medication
Reminders:
High cholesterol
BP check needed
Last consultation:
Three weeks ago, for general health check and discussion of a variety of health issues – hair loss, ankle sprain, hay fever and plantar fasciitis.

Patient view

Mr NA is a successful businessman who does a lot of travelling and entertaining in his job. He doesn't have time for regular exercise, but he wants to do whatever he can to stay healthy.

I ordered some routine blood tests for him two weeks ago, and he has been asked to come in to discuss the results. He has been told that his cholesterol is raised. His blood pressure was also high last time so that needs checking again. He has had to take time out of his busy day to come to the doctor's (for the second time in two weeks) so he also wants to get his foot sorted, which is no better since last time.

The trouble with preventing illness is that if I am doing my job well, nothing much should happen. I sometimes envy the surgeons who go in, take out, or mend bits – when everything's sewn up, they have something to show for their work. Offending morsel removed, pain sorted, blockage cleared, signed off with a neat scar. For me, success means no heart attack, no stroke, not developing diabetes. There's nothing much to see.

It may not be as sexy as surgery, but in terms of healthy lives saved, the evidence says our preventive work is just as important. And it can be professionally rewarding; for instance when a patient bounces in who you just know, if medicine hadn't intervened, should have died or had a stroke years earlier.

Preventing illness and disease is now a huge chunk of a GP's work. Even twenty-five years ago when I was a trainee, checking blood pressure was a rather haphazard activity. And if it was high, doing something about it was even more hit-or-miss. I don't think we fully understood the importance of keeping blood pressure low, or cholesterol under control – at least it wasn't a priority. We didn't even measure cholesterol when I was training. When you consider that roughly half of the ten leading causes of death in the UK can be traced to lifestyle and behaviour, it's just as well that preventive medicine has become a special focus in primary care. As a GP I take pride in my unique expertise in this area.

Mr NA looks a bit like me. He's a big man, carrying more poundage than he should, but not Michelin Man fat. I saw him a couple of weeks ago when he presented me with a list of problems to sort out. The appointment felt more like a business meeting than a consultation with the doctor. One of the tasks he gave me was to give him a 'health check' because he is now in his late fifties and hasn't had a proper health 'MOT' before. He wasn't quite sure what he wanted checking, but cholesterol and the 'prostate cancer' blood test were two requests that cropped up. Now he's back for the results.

Everything was normal except that his cholesterol is pretty high – 6.8. Blood cholesterol is measured in units called millimoles per litre of blood, often shortened to mmol/L. The UK government recommends that total cholesterol levels should be 5 mmol/L or less for healthy adults, or 4 mmol/L or less for those at high risk. The evidence suggests that in fact the lower it is, the better. Cholesterol is essential for lots of our body's functions, from maintaining healthy cell membranes to making crucial hormones and vitamins – but when it's high it can start to build up in your artery walls, restricting the blood flow to your heart, your brain and the rest of your body.

I also measured NA's blood pressure (BP) last time and it was raised at 160/98. The evidence-based guidelines say his BP should be below 140/90 – again, the lower the better, so long as you don't keep falling over or feeling dizzy.

'So we're talking about your blood results today, that's right, isn't it?'

'Yes, apparently my cholesterol's high. Now I know why that is – my diet's been terrible recently. Meals out, entertaining and so on. So I'm sure I can get it lower very easily. How high was it actually?'

'Quite high. It came back as 6.8. We like it below 5 – or even lower if possible.'

The last time I measured my own cholesterol, it was 5.9. The old joke goes that the medical definition of an alcoholic is someone who drinks more than their doctor; in the same way, I confess I find it hard to get worked up by a cholesterol level that's not much higher than my own.

'Does anyone in your family have high cholesterol?'

I'm thinking of a condition called familial hypercholesterolaemia – about 1 in 500 people inherit from one of their parents a genetic defect that means they have higher levels of LDL cholesterol ('bad' cholesterol), which increases the risk of heart attacks and strokes at an early age, say before fifty. Usually familial hypercholesterolaemia pushes the total cholesterol up to around 7.5 though, so it's unlikely here.

'Not that I know of.'

'And I think I asked last time, but has anyone in the family suffered a heart attack or stroke at an early age?'

When it comes to assessing someone's risk for heart disease or stroke, there's a strong genetic component. Even if you don't have familial hypercholesterolaemia, we know your genes influence your cholesterol levels, blood pressure and risk of diabetes to some extent.

All of these are important risk factors for heart disease and stroke. And if a first-degree blood relative has had coronary heart disease or stroke before the age of fifty-five years (for a male relative) or sixty-five years (for a female relative), your risk increases. If both your parents have suffered from heart disease before the age of fifty-five, your risk of developing heart disease can rise by 50 per cent compared to the general population. I am aware of your ethnicity here too – for example, South Asian people living in the UK are about one and a half times more likely to die from coronary heart disease before the age of seventy-five than the rest of the UK population.

'My older brother is fine. Father died of cancer in his seventies. Mother's still alive – she has diabetes.'

'OK. Let's talk numbers.'

I am aware that I am mimicking his straight-talking style. It can be helpful to adapt my communication style to the patient in front of me – particularly when we are talking about attitudes to health risks. For some people, I might try to find a suitable analogy to set out the risks (for example, the pressure in a central heating system or a hosepipe, or the build-up of debris on the sides of a drain), but I get the sense that NA would find that patronising, and wants to get to the point. I swivel the computer screen around so that we can look at the data together.

'The total cholesterol level itself is high – 6.9. Then we break that down into HDL ("good" cholesterol) and LDL ("bad" cholesterol) – do you know about that?'

'Yes, I've heard of it.'

'So your HDL – here – is roughly normal, but your LDL – here – is high. So your overall cholesterol is high, and of that, it's mostly the damaging LDL sort.'

'Right, right. But that's something I can correct, is it?'

'Well, you say that there's room for improvement on the diet side – that would certainly help. Cutting down on saturated fats (like fatty meats, hard cheese, butter or cream) and replacing them with small amounts of unsaturated fats (like vegetable oil or oily fish) – can help. We should be avoiding trans fats too (in things like fried foods, take-aways, biscuits, cakes or pastries). Worth eating more fibre as well – that can help reduce your cholesterol; fruit and vegetables, wholemeal bread and so on. I can give you a leaflet about that. We also know that doing more exercise and losing weight, if you have any to lose, can help lower cholesterol. Do you think you have any weight to lose?'

Recently I have rather taken to that phrase 'Do you think you have any weight to lose?', or something similar. In years gone by, the doctor would more often than not tell the patient what they needed to do: lose some weight, stop smoking, take these pills, take up golf and so on. The trouble is that patients just don't do as they are told. Even in the face of overwhelming evidence, if we get a response at all, it's often 'Yes, but'. Not only has the relationship between doctor and patient become less paternalistic (I can't think of many modern patients who'd take kindly to being told what to do), but the evidence clearly suggests that telling people what to do rarely works. If you have a toddler or a teenager, you'll really understand.

Like most GPs, I am now much more likely to use a technique called motivational interviewing to help people change their behaviour. It was first developed in the 1980s as a way to help people with problem drinking and other addictions, but it can be used for all sorts of situations where changing behaviour is the goal. The idea is to guide the patient and tap into their own motivation for change. It's a non-judgemental approach, much more about supporting people than telling them off. The key ingredients of motivational interviewing can be summed up in the acronym RULE. R is about **R**esisting the 'righting reflex' – the urge to set things right and tell people what they should or shouldn't do. Instead, recognising that you may have doubts about whether you want to change, and whether you are able to do so, I need to help you weigh up the pros and cons. U stands for **U**nderstanding the patient's own motivations. What are their experiences so far, what has or hasn't worked for them? L is about **L**istening with empathy, and E is about **E**mpowering the patient, encouraging hope and optimism.

So I tend to use questions like 'Do you think you have any weight to lose?' or 'What do you think might be stopping you from losing weight?' or 'What has worked best for you in the past?' If you want to motivate someone, a question like 'How would things change for you if you were able to lose a couple of kilograms?' is more likely to be helpful than 'You really should lose some weight, you know.'

There's another model of behaviour change that GPs sometimes use in helping people to change health behaviours. Prochaska and DiClemente's 'stages of change' model describes the stages people go through on their journey to changing behaviour. They start in a pre-contemplation stage – they're not ready to change anything yet, and they're not planning on any action. The next stage is the contemplation stage – getting ready for action. They're weighing up the pros and cons, but they haven't made up their mind. GPs spend a lot of time trying to shift people from the pre-contemplation stage to the contemplation stage. Motivational interviewing can really help with the next three stages of the model – preparation (getting ready), action (making specific changes) and maintenance (trying to prevent relapse).

Having said all that, sometimes patients just need (and want) a kick up the bum. Given the right sort of relationship (something we can develop in primary care), a well-aimed boot in the pants can be very effective.

'Well I suppose I could lose a few pounds, yes.'

'OK, so what do you think would work best for you to lose some weight – any room for some more physical activity?'

'I used to play a lot of rugby, but gave up – broken collar bone, getting too old. I like cycling, could do more of that; maybe cycle to work more often.'

He's lost in thought now; his eyes would be staring off into the trees at the end of the leafy suburban garden behind me, if the blind was up. It's what Roger Neighbour calls the 'internal search', like a do-not-disturb sign. I shut up and let him do his mental homework.

'. . . or walking the dog – could certainly do more of that.'

'Great, well, I think that could all certainly make a difference. Well worth the effort.'

(*two minutes*)

I've heard people say that doctors should practise what they preach – doctors shouldn't be overweight. But we are human and fallible like everyone else, and actually I think there may even be a plus side to being a lardy middle-aged doctor: I can empathise with patients who struggle to lose weight. That doesn't mean I'm soft – I am very clear about the risks a patient is taking by being overweight and the benefits of shedding some avoirdupois. But it does mean I really understand the challenges. On the one hand it is straightforward – eat less and move more. A simple equation – burn off more calories than you consume. The scientist in me gets irritated by very overweight people who claim to 'eat like a bird' or have 'glandular problems'. Some people are even more impatient, their intolerance of obesity being based on a shocking logical leap – that there were no fat people in Belsen.

Apart from the ethical ugliness of that comparison, losing weight by force in a concentration camp is of course entirely different from maintaining a healthy weight in modern society. The modern obesity epidemic is a complex problem. We live in an obesogenic environment. Weight is influenced by a huge range of social, political, psychological (often), and (occasionally) discrete physical problems like thyroid disorders, or exercise-limiting arthritis. Genetic factors play a part too – our genes may affect the amount of body fat we store, where that fat is distributed, and how efficiently the body converts food into energy. I am sure my own weight struggles are tied up with my very sedentary job; emotional baggage which leads me to see food as a great comfort when I am anxious, sad or exhausted; ready access to tasty high-calorie foods and drinks that I wasn't allowed when I was younger; and a sense of lack of time. I can probably even blame a few pounds on my genes too – family legend tells of a 40-stone blacksmith ancestor (I'm not quite there yet). I try to be active – I cycle to work, run round the park every week, walk the dog every day, and every few months I'll try some system of eating much less (I've done the 5:2 diet, the cabbage soup diet; weight-watching groups; and branded diet drinks to name a few – all of them worked . . . for a bit). But there's still a thin person inside me, screaming to get out.

Of course the answer is that I need to eat less and exercise more for the long term – and that is down to me. But there are some notable barriers standing in the way. I also used to smoke cigarettes, and what helped me kick that habit was clear information about the health risks (as a doctor, I was pretty *au fait* with those; at medical school we were only allowed to smoke in the pathology museum, surrounded by bottled specimens of lung cancer), help with clarifying my motivation to stop (especially the benefits of stopping, not the harms of continuing), understanding the barriers, and empathetic support. In the end I got that from our local pharmacist, who runs an excellent stop-smoking service. It wasn't the repeated bossy or anxious calls for action I had over the years from family, friends, or doctors. I had to be ready – really motivated – to stop. And then I needed support. I hope that experience makes me better able to help others to stop.

'Of course having high cholesterol isn't a disease in itself – it's just one of several risk factors for developing heart disease or stroke. These days we can actually estimate your risk of going on to develop heart disease or stroke, based on all the risk factors we know about. So we feed in whether you smoke or not, whether you have diabetes, any family history, your cholesterol, your blood pressure, your BMI and so on, and the computer works out your percentage risk of developing heart disease or stroke over the next ten years.'

This is usually a great way to focus the mind – most people want to know their risk of having a heart attack or stroke in the next ten years. AN's eyes are like lasers pointing at the screen, willing me to get on with it . . .

'And here you are: 16 per cent risk over the next ten years. Now, when your risk goes over 20 per cent (that's a one in five chance), the balance swings in favour of considering medication to lower your cholesterol. In fact the latest guidance suggests I should offer statins to anyone with a risk above just 10 per cent (a one in ten chance). Do you know much about statins?'

It's a dumb question really. Most of my patients know all about statins – the single most commonly prescribed class of treatment in the developed world, taken by tens if not hundreds of millions of patients every day. I sometimes suspect that they're the main topic of conversation among the over-sixties in my neck of the woods. They work mainly by reducing the production of cholesterol in the liver, but they may also help your body reabsorb cholesterol that has built up on your artery walls, preventing further blockage in your blood vessels and heart attacks.

There is good-quality trial evidence that statins reduce death rates from all causes, and from cardiovascular disease, and the size of the benefit is greater for those with the greatest risk. It's possible that some of their beneficial effects may be related more to their anti-inflammatory properties or the functioning of the lining of blood vessels than to their cholesterol-lowering action. But many of my patients don't trust statins – they read in the papers or hear from friends about side effects. Actually, most people who take statins don't get any side effects, but a small minority do complain of problems like fatigue, headache, nausea, indigestion, mood changes or change in bowel habit. Statins have also been linked to an increased risk of developing diabetes. Probably the most debated side effect is what's called myalgia – muscle aches and pains. Side effects, and stopping statins because of them, are fairly common. But for some it's hard to be sure that statins are to blame. In fact one recent study, which reviewed lots of randomised placebo-controlled trials of statins, came to the conclusion that only a small minority of symptoms reported on statins are genuinely due to the statins: almost all would occur just as frequently on a placebo. Extremely rarely – affecting less than 1 in 10,000 people – statins can cause a breakdown of the muscle cells, a serious condition known as rhabdomyolysis.

Though using statins in people at high risk of stroke and heart disease is uncontroversial, recent recommendations by the National Institute of Health and Care Excellence (NICE) suggested that we should start offering statins to our outwardly healthy, low-risk patients. It set the cat among the pigeons, triggering the so-called 'statin wars'. The NICE standpoint, based on updated evidence, was that statins should now be considered to prevent cardiovascular disease even in people at low risk – in other words those with a one in ten (10 per cent) risk over the next ten years rather than just those with a one in five (20 per cent) risk. For some horrified doctors who wrote a letter to the Health Secretary to express their concerns, that meant condemning most healthy middle-aged adults to lifelong medications of questionable value and possible side effects. They questioned the evidence on which the new guidance was based – mostly studies funded by the pharmaceutical industry. They worried about the creeping medicalisation of modern society; turning healthy people into patients and potentially causing more harm than good. One cardiologist made the point that although there is good evidence that the benefits of statins outweigh the potential harms in those with established heart disease, this is clearly not the case for healthy people at low risk. He compared it to giving insulin to someone who doesn't have diabetes, or chemotherapy to someone without cancer. There's growing momentum in raising awareness of the problem of medicalisation – not just with regard to the widespread use of statins, but also for example, with over-prescribing of antibiotics, or over-diagnosing mildly raised blood pressure or pre-diabetes. The pros and cons of the statin argument rumble on, and it's fair to say that the US guidelines take a similar line. And NICE has always made it clear that this needs to be an individual decision, after trying lifestyle changes, and after carefully balancing the pros and cons. But I am not alone as a GP in being worried about the dangers of 'too much medicine' – over-diagnosis, over-treatment, and the creeping medicalisation of modern society.

It can be frustrating as a doctor when your patients seem to be unimpressed by your explanations; for example, when you're convinced by strong evidence from trials that treatment A is much more effective than treatment B. Often, media reports and chats with friends seem to carry more sway. Our trial evidence is often based on data from huge populations. My job now is to somehow explain, in a fair and clear way, what that means for the individual patient sitting in front of me. This is where I become more like a financial adviser than a doctor. My adviser gets me to fill out a questionnaire to find out my attitudes to investment risk before advising one product or another.

Of course, there are times when clinicians *have* to make decisions for their patients – in emergencies, when patients are unconscious or for other reasons don't have capacity to make decisions for themselves.

And sometimes patients ask me, 'What would you do, doc?' But since the 1980s, the idea of sharing decision making with patients has gained increasing prominence. Research suggests that most patients want to be involved in decisions about their care. There's also mounting evidence to suggest that shared decision making is a 'good thing' – it leads to better consultations, clearer risk communication, improved health literacy, fewer unwanted treatments, healthier lifestyles, improved confidence and self-efficacy, safer care, reduced costs and better health outcomes.

But in practice, the challenge of teaching doctors about shared decision making is that people make decisions based on more than just facts. It's so tempting to throw the scientific evidence at the patient, like giving them a jab with a giant data syringe, and expect them to make the same decision as you would. But personal values play such a crucial role in decision making – and people's values are influenced by all sorts of factors; their personal experiences, their ethics, their religion or cultural background. Different patients, faced with the same choices and the same evidence, may make very different decisions. Not right or wrong decisions – just different ones, right for them. What's important for me (and my students or trainees) to grasp is that my values as a doctor may be very different to my patient's values. So when I am helping patients make decisions, understanding and taking account of the patient's values is as important as all the number talk.

So what will NA put up with now, to offer him the possibility of a modest reduction in the risk of heart attacks and strokes many years down the line? I explain that he will need to be on statins for ever – if he stops, he stops the benefit. There's a small risk of side effects too – though they are usually reversible, and we can always reduce the dose or have a break to see if it helps. He'll need to avoid taking them at the same time as some other medications and, bizarrely, grapefruit juice (the latter prevents enzymes in the body from breaking down statins, so statin levels can increase, which makes side effects more likely). We'll need to do blood tests to check his liver is OK – statins can affect liver function too.

When it comes to explaining the benefit, I can now use software that takes account of his individual risk, and creates a visual representation of the potential benefits using pictures of 100 or 1000 people. It's a simplistic model, but I find it easier to understand, even if the patient doesn't always.

'So, if we imagine 100 people with exactly the same level of risk as you – 16 per cent. Without statins, this many – the ones coloured red – will have a heart attack or stroke over the next ten years. And this many – coloured green – will have their heart attack or stroke prevented, because they are taking statins. And this many – coloured orange – will have a heart attack or stroke regardless of whether they are on statins or not.'

He's following me – the pictorial approach does make it clearer. Of course it is a simplified version, and can't be exactly matched to any individual, but it's the best evidence we have, delivered in the clearest way I can manage in a ten-minute consultation.

'Look, I don't think I'll start the statins. I've heard too many problems about them, and it looks like it's a small gain anyway. I know I can change my diet, and that should make a difference. I'd rather try that first.'

'OK, that's fine.' I'm quite relieved.

(four minutes)

'Can we recheck your cholesterol in, say, six months' time in that case, to see how you're doing on the diet?' I enter a request for a repeat fasting blood test in six months. That just means he needs to avoid eating anything for ten to twelve hours before the blood test so that his LDL cholesterol levels aren't influenced too much by what he has just digested. There's a newer type of cholesterol test that doesn't involve fasting. It measures non-high density lipoprotein (non-HDL) because that's thought to be more accurate in estimating cardiovascular disease (CVD) risk than LDL. Non-HDL cholesterol is just the total cholesterol minus the HDL cholesterol (though strangely, that's not the same as LDL cholesterol).

I know from experience, and from the research literature, that improving the diet can help but it's rarely enough to drop cholesterol significantly – unless the diet is really terrible. Cream teas, biscuits, cakes, cheese, loads of red meat – a bit like my diet on a hangover day. For most people (with a few notable exceptions) any reduction in cholesterol from changes in diet alone is usually modest – and that depends on sticking to it. But I am happy to go along with his plans. I have done my duty – explained the risks and benefits, and given him some material to read. I now make a careful record in the notes that we have discussed the pros and cons and the patient has decided not to take statins for now. I have been glad of that in the past, for example when a patient had a heart attack, and a relative complained that I had not treated his blood pressure properly (the hospital doctors had helpfully pointed out that the blood pressure was very 'poorly controlled', which was the cause of the heart attack). In fact I had had several conversations offering blood pressure medications, strongly recommending them, which the patient had declined. Fortunately, I had recorded those discussions in the notes.

The most important modifiable risk factors for heart disease and strokes are smoking, high cholesterol, high blood pressure, being overweight and inactive, and having diabetes. Then, in division two, there's stress, drinking too much alcohol, and a poor diet. Stopping smoking is probably the most important single lifestyle change to reduce risk. I didn't mind putting on a bit of weight when I stopped smoking – the risks of smoking far outweigh the risks of being a bit overweight. Mr NA doesn't smoke – if he did, I would enjoy showing him the effect of stopping smoking on his percentage risk. Type in 'non-smoker' instead of 'smoker', press the return key with a flourish, and hey presto: the percentage risk tumbles by roughly half.

So I've tackled cholesterol, weight, diet and exercise – at least as much as is practicable in the time. Now I need to turn to his blood pressure, which was raised last time. I can't reliably diagnose high blood pressure on the basis of one reading – one-off readings are notoriously unreliable. For a start, blood pressure varies throughout the day – it's normally lower at night while you're sleeping, starts to rise a few hours before you wake up, and then continues to rise during the day, usually peaking in the middle of the afternoon. Then in the late afternoon and evening, your blood pressure begins dropping again. There's also the problem of the so-called 'white coat effect'. This is a phenomenon affecting up to one in five adults, in which blood pressure measurements taken at your doctor's or in a clinic are high, even though your blood pressure's normal the rest of the time. Bizarrely, it's not just about anxiety.

So I need at least three readings – or better still, these days the recommendation is that we either get patients to monitor their own blood pressure at home over a set period (using a properly calibrated machine), or we ask them to wear a blood pressure monitor for twenty-four hours. I feel happier with the twenty-four-hour monitoring – it seems more objective to me – but it can be quite intrusive. The cuff suddenly pumps itself up around your arm every half hour or so, perhaps during an important meeting, and it keeps doing that throughout the night.

I check NA's blood pressure today, and it's still up, even after we leave it a few minutes and take it again without chatting while we do so (that can raise it too). I've used the large arm cuff too – too small a cuff will falsely increase the BP readings.

(*eight minutes*)

'Look, it's still raised: 165/99. I think the best thing to do would be to check your blood pressure over twenty-four hours – that gives the most reliable readings. Now, that does mean wearing a monitoring device for twenty-four hours – it pumps itself up every half an hour – even in the night – but if you can bear it, it'll give us the most accurate readings and we can decide what to do then.'

'Yes, OK. I'd rather get it sorted. I can't for the life of me understand why I have high blood pressure though. It's always been absolutely fine.'

'Well, high blood pressure is partly down to our genes – so we're just made that way . . . the blood pressure rises as we get older. The other main causes would be excess alcohol, too much salt in the diet, and being overweight. Any of those apply?'

We work out he drinks about thirty units of alcohol a week – probably an underestimate. He doesn't feel it's too much, but the current national guidelines for men (fourteen units a week) would disagree.

'I just drink socially – not a huge amount at all.' People often think that drinking socially doesn't really count, as if the alcohol content is diluted if you share it with other people.

His diet includes a lot of eating out and he does add salt to his food as well. I don't have time now to explore his alcohol habits any deeper, and I get the sense that he doesn't want to either. But I spell out the guidance, and explain the link to high blood pressure.

One of the great challenges of treating blood pressure is that most people don't have any symptoms from it at all. It affects roughly a quarter of the British adult population and accounts for 60 per cent of all strokes in the UK and half of all heart attacks, but because it's usually symptomless most people have no idea they are at risk until it is too late. The cliché 'silent killer' really does apply here. I need to scare NA sufficiently for him to take notice, without him shutting down completely, figuratively covering his ears with both hands and shouting 'la la la' over me.

I must move on now. I shift into 'telling' mode. I know we're trained to share management plans with patients, and check they are happy and so on, but, right now, just telling him what's going to happen is quicker. And I think he prefers it given to him straight.

'Look, book yourself in for a twenty-four-hour BP monitor at the front desk and then come and see me with those results to discuss what to do next. It might show that your blood pressure is actually fine. And if not, we have other options up our sleeve – from changing diet, exercise and cutting down alcohol a bit, to thinking about medications if they're needed.'

'I'm not one for pills. I wouldn't be keen to take pills at all.'

Me neither. Of course, if we can avoid them, we will. Medicalisation and all that. But in a modern GP surgery, medicines are going to be on the menu. If I was given a penny for every time a patient said they weren't 'really one for pills' I'd be a millionaire. It always seems to me a bit like going to the butcher's and saying 'I'm not really one for meat'.

'OK?' I say, meaning 'Is that everything?'

(*ten minutes*)

'Oh, while I'm here – my feet. I've been doing the exercises and stretches but they're really no better. It's absolutely killing me. Is there an injection or something?'

'While I'm here' is another phrase you get used to as a GP. It used to wind me up, but now I just smile inside and count to ten.

We discussed this the last time he came, but there was a long list to address then, and probably much of what we said didn't sink in. So I go over it again.

Plantar fasciitis is a painful condition affecting the sole of the foot, especially around the heel. The plantar fascia is a thick band of tough tissue, like a ligament, that runs along the sole of your foot from your heel to your middle foot bones. The fascia can become inflamed (anything ending in -*itis* just means inflammation, hence *fasciitis*) and painful, especially if you are on your feet a lot, or running or walking more than usual. It goes in time (often a few months) and, as with lots of musculoskeletal problems, the best we can do is relieve symptoms and help the body to heal itself as quickly as possible. In other words, the approach is rest, good footwear, heel pads, anti-inflammatories, and stretching exercises of various sorts. In more severe cases, and if these conservative approaches don't do the trick after a decent length of time, sometimes we try a steroid injection – but it's a painful procedure. It may relieve the pain for some people for a few weeks, but it doesn't always cure the problem so sometimes you need several injections. And steroid injections are not without their risks – in this case, for example, the small risk of rupturing the fascia itself.

I am empathetic, well aware that plantar fasciitis can be very painful. But although NA wants a quick fix so he can get on with his busy life, I am not convinced that a steroid injection is in his best interests. Sometimes I have to push the conservative approach to save the patient from themselves – the body is amazing at healing itself and it's usually best left to do the job naturally in its own time, however inconvenient or unsatisfying that may be. For someone like NA, now's a time to be quite directive.

'Look, as I said, it is something that should settle down with time; and the injections are painful, they don't always cure the problem, and they do carry risks. If you want my advice, I'd give it a bit longer. You are doing all the right things. We can always keep the injections up our sleeve if things aren't settling over the next few weeks. What do you think?'

'OK, we'll see how it goes. Can I call you if it's not getting better?'

'Leave a message for me at reception and I'll ring you back . . . the option is always there if you feel strongly about it.'

'OK, right you are.'

I rise from my chair with a 'Thanks for coming in . . .' It's the GP's equivalent of the bartender's 'Time gentlemen, please'. He understands.

(*twelve minutes*)

Chapter 5

Mr EK

(running thirteen minutes late)

Doctor view

Appointment time: 8.10
Name: Mr EK
Age: 36 years old
Occupation: Unemployed builder
Past medical history:
 No record
Medication:
 Citalopram (antidepressant)
Reminders:
 None
Last consultation:
 One week ago, for a first episode of depression; started antidepressants and referred for counselling. This is a planned review one week later.

Patient view

Mr EK came to the UK from Eastern Europe last year and he is struggling. He lives on his own in a tiny flat, he is single, and he can't get work as a builder. His English is poor. He has family back in Belarus who he is worried about, and misses, and at the moment life looks bleak. He is desperately lonely and London has not lived up to its promise.

He understands he is not well; but he cannot see a way out of his situation at all, apart from possibly killing himself, which he has thought about quite a lot recently.

The pills the doctor gave him last time don't seem to be working at all, and the counselling is not going to happen for another month at the earliest. He is not impressed.

When I was thirteen, I saw a woman jump in front of a high-speed train. I was on my way home from school, standing on the platform. Opposite me, just a few feet across the tracks, was a middle-aged lady clutching a plastic hold-all bag. I don't remember her face, but she was holding tight onto the bag in front of her with both hands, shuffling slowly to the edge of her platform as the tracks started to sing. The metallic hiss grew closer, louder. The guard, my side, clapped his hands and shouted at her to move back from the edge. But she stuck, robot-like, to her plan. She jumped down onto the tracks and crouched, with her bag, waiting. She was hunched there for a second or two before the train struck her. After the train, there was just blood, body parts and her bag.

I remember everyone on the platform wailing. I couldn't bear to look at the blood on the tracks, so I edged around to the other side of the little waiting room on the platform and stood stiff with my back stuck to the wall, eyes closed, like a fugitive hiding from a search party. When I finally got on my own train home, some passengers quizzed me on the details. What had happened? What did it look like? Was it a high-speed train? How did she do it exactly? A kind man next to me told them to leave me alone – couldn't they see I was in shock? For many years I felt guilty that I hadn't jumped down onto the tracks in those couple of seconds as she froze there, and hauled her to safety.

But what disturbed me most was not the guilt or the gore. It was the shocking realisation that anyone could do that to themselves at all. It was hard for a thirteen-year-old boy to conceive of that kind of despair, that sense of hopelessness. It still intrigues and drives me now – the goings-on in the minds of people with mental illness. Some GPs find dealing with emotional and psychological problems very difficult. It's rarely easy, but I am a GP who enjoys the challenge of delving into someone's psyche and trying to find a way to understand, clarify, even help. I often think of that poor woman when I see people like Mr EK.

When he came last week, he worried me. He was clearly depressed and told me he often thought he might be better off dead; that would at least put an end to his problems. I've been thinking about him a lot since we met. I have felt concerned that in the fifteen minutes we shared last week, I wasn't able to answer adequately his desperate, brave plea for help. There was a painful moment over breakfast one day too, when my daughter, who was excitedly telling me about her dance show, realised I wasn't listening to her at all. My eyes were looking in her direction, but she saw that they were focused elsewhere. She was right – I was not with her in that instant. I was with EK, alone in his dismal flat, weighing up the pros and cons of ending it all.

When I say EK was obviously depressed, I mean that you would probably have come to that conclusion, whether you are medically trained or not. All the signs were there. He was tearful, and he seemed distant, somehow disconnected. It was hard to make proper eye contact with him as he was always gazing at his shoes. He whiffed like he hadn't washed for more than a week and his clothes were grubby and thrown together: the self-neglect of someone who has lost a sense of purpose in life. His speech was monotonous and slow, and his sentences often trailed off. For illnesses of the mind, my examination focuses on these sorts of features. We call it a mental state examination. Unlike a physical examination, which is usually clearly signposted and separate from the history-taking phase of the consultation, my mental state examination is going on at the same time as I am gathering specific information from the patient's history.

I'm particularly scanning EK's appearance, body language, speech and mood. In more severe psychiatric illness, there may be psychotic features such as either visual or auditory hallucinations, delusions and paranoid thoughts, alongside a loss of insight. About half of people living with schizophrenia, and a smaller percentage of those who live with bipolar disorder (who may present with depression), sometimes don't realise that they have a psychiatric illness. The medical term for not seeing what's wrong with you is anosognosia, or a lack of insight. It's not that they are 'in denial', it is really a part of the illness – it's probably that the frontal lobes in their brain (which are needed for interpreting experiences) aren't working as they should. I have only come across people with full-blown psychotic features a handful of times in general practice – mostly people with schizophrenia or mania – but it is something I learned about and dealt with a lot in the hospital phase of my training. I need to recognise it when I see it, and I'm always on the look-out for it.

GPs see about one depressed patient every surgery, but they don't all walk in saying 'I'm feeling depressed.' People often mention that they are lacking in energy, or focus on a very physical symptom such as generalised body aches and pains or headaches. Occasionally the physical symptoms surface as bizarre neurological features such as involuntary movements, a feeling of a lump in the throat, or even seizures. I have to take these at face value – the first step is always to exclude any physical problems. For example, a sensation of a lump in the throat used to be called globus hystericus because it was thought that it was a sign of hysteria – mental illness particularly linked to 'disturbances of the uterus' (from the Greek for uterus – *hystera*). But nowadays we know we need to make sure it's not a problem with the nerve supply to the oesophagus (gullet), a problem with the complex coordination of muscles during swallowing, something stuck in the throat, acid reflux irritating the gullet, or even a cancer.

But when those investigations come back normal, and the discussions veer into psychological territory, things can get tricky. Some people are open to the suggestion that what they are experiencing may be related to underlying psychological problems, and that can be extremely rewarding for them and for me. But sometimes it goes down like a fart in a spacesuit. The stigma around mental illness, which probably contributes to its transformation into physical problems in the first place, can also make people very reluctant to entertain the possibility that their physical symptoms might have a psychological origin.

'Are you saying it's all in my mind, Doctor?'

I'm not saying that at all. I am acknowledging that the mind is extremely powerful and it can often trigger very real physical symptoms in all of us. When we feel anxious we start to sweat, our heart beats faster, we might shake. So perhaps rather than organising yet another scan or yet another blood test or seeing yet another specialist in search of the Holy Grail of a physical diagnostic label, I genuinely believe that the patient sometimes may get better faster if we explore the psychological. The trouble is that you can never say never in medicine. (I learned this early on in medical school exams: for example, if a multiple choice question says 'A *never* causes B', it's almost certainly wrong.) So I am trying to be at my most persuasive by suggesting a psychological root, while also keeping the door open to the remote possibility that the physical symptoms might, after all, be caused by an organic disease despite all the tests coming back 'normal'. It happens.

So in many ways it is a relief to see EK, who has fairly 'straightforward' clinical depression. He told me he was depressed. When I explored how he was feeling last week, he outlined perfectly the difference between feeling sad (a normal part of human existence) and being clinically depressed (a debilitating mental illness). I have been clinically depressed myself – twice I think, once as a medical student, and once more recently. It is absolutely not a feeling of sadness – your thinking is too blunted to feel 'sad'. Your mood is not focused on anything in particular. It is more painful than any physical pain I have experienced – an overwhelming absence of pleasure in anything. I felt a kind of numbness that made me seem detached from the outside world, deeply alone, and for me the only escape was sleep. When I awoke, I just wanted to go back to sleep again. It was very hard to see the point in anything, including myself, and I could not see a way out.

If someone comes to me feeling like that, it's likely that they are going to struggle to express themselves eloquently. I certainly wasn't able to. Nevertheless, we doctors are trained to find out whether someone has 'lost interest and enjoyment' in the things they would normally enjoy (called anhedonia, another echo of medicine's Greek roots), or whether they have a sense of 'worthlessness or guilt' or 'hopelessness'. As words, they don't seem to be quite enough.

We are much more proactive about depression than we were ten years ago. There are two particular questions that I sometimes ask as screening questions for depression, often in people who are at high risk (for example, those with chronic diseases or cancers, or those with difficult social issues). Research suggests that out of 100 patients with depression these two questions should pick up 96 of them:

1. 'During the last month, have you often been bothered by feeling down, depressed or hopeless?'
2. 'During the last month, have you often been bothered by little interest or pleasure in doing things?'

I also sometimes ask patients to complete a more formal questionnaire, called the PHQ-9 (Patient Health Questionnaire-9), which helps with the diagnosis and can be useful in grading depression as mild, moderate or severe. These sorts of questionnaires can be helpful in picking up depression, or monitoring changes over time, and they offer some kind of comforting measurability for a condition that can be hard to pin down. But the great danger of this tick-box medicine is that it reduces what the patient is feeling to a set of numbers and can turn what should be a therapeutic human interaction into a mechanistic survey.

For 'straightforward' depression, where the patient retains insight into his condition, and there are no psychotic signs, the history is all important. So I start with an open question, inviting EK to describe things in his own words:

'Thanks for coming back today. So how are you feeling?'

I emphasise the word *feeling*, and I think I am wearing a slight frown of concern. This should not be the 'How are you?' you might say to someone at the bus stop, when a detailed reply would be an unexpected imposition. I really *do* want him to tell me how he's feeling.

'Not good.' He is staring at the floor.

When you're depressed, your thinking gets sluggish, your concentration wavers, and your speech can soften and slow down. He is sucking me into his slow-motion world, and in order to connect with him, I need to meet him there. I need to be ready for longer silences, softer speech: time will slow down and there's no point in me trying to speed it up. I just need to make sure that it doesn't leave me feeling depressed – a recognised phenomenon.

I leave a longer than normal silence, picking up the rhythm of the exchange. Then I say, softly: 'In what way, not good?'

'Just . . . Not good . . . Crying . . .'

'You're still crying a lot, are you?'

'Yes. And not sleeping.' He is weeping now, tears tumbling from his cheeks onto the floor. I leave some space.

'I'm sorry to hear that. What's the worst thing about this for you?'

I listen again at length about the gaps, the absences, the disappointments and the loneliness. No family, no job, no language, no friends.

Anyone would struggle, and I feel for him. What would help most? Right now he may need a doctor, but at the heart of it, he needs his family, some friends, a job, and some English. I can't conjure that lot up on prescription. How can I really help?

I fall back on the comforting routine of the psychiatric history.

(four minutes)

EK may remember me asking him last week the key questions I have to ask all people with depression or anxiety (they often go hand in hand). These are questions about some of the biological symptoms which frequently accompany depression. For example, sleep problems – particularly trouble getting off to sleep, or waking up early and not being able to get back to sleep. People often describe difficulty concentrating too. Changes in weight or appetite is another:

'Has your appetite changed at all?' Depressed people often lose their appetite – or the opposite – they start to over-eat.

'I'm not eating much, no.'

'And what about your weight – any change there?'

'No, it's the same. Doctor, please can you help me? The pills are not working.'

I'm aware that I am asking lots of questions here; that's important, but ultimately there is huge therapeutic value in listening, witnessing, empathising, and offering some hope. It's what psychoanalyst Michael Balint called using the 'doctor as drug'. Most UK GPs will know about Balint – he began a seminal discussion and support group for family doctors and his work contributed many useful concepts to our understanding of the doctor–patient relationship. One of them was to highlight the therapeutic power of the doctor him or herself, apart from the treatments they prescribe. I can help – now it's time to tap into that doctor drug.

'Look, you are clinically depressed at the moment – that is a deeply unpleasant illness, and right now it must seem like there is no light at the end of the tunnel. But believe me – you will get better from this; it may take a little time, but we will help you and support you and you will feel yourself again.'

I'm aware that might sound a little too sanguine, and I suspect that in his present state he will struggle to believe me. But he gently nods; I read it as a grateful gesture.

'Right – well, as we talked about last week, the pills do sometimes take a couple of weeks or more to start working properly. Have you had any side effects from them?'

'No, I don't think so.'

(*five minutes*)

Last week, I referred him for talking therapy, and pointed him to self-help materials and mental health charities in the meantime (despite a recent push to improve access to psychological therapies like counselling, I know he won't actually be seen for twelve weeks or so). I also started him on 20 mg of Citalopram. That's a Selective Serotonin Reuptake Inhibitor or SSRI – a modern member of the Prozac family of antidepressants. SSRIs increase the concentration of the 'happy hormone' serotonin – a chemical messenger within the nervous system. The theory goes that a deficiency in the normal working of serotonin in the central nervous system is the cause of, or a predisposing factor for, depression. However, the evidence for this association is largely circumstantial and it certainly doesn't explain everything about depression – there are probably multiple factors at play. Some trials also cast doubt on how effective SSRIs are compared with a placebo. But despite this, antidepressants are still useful for about half of people with moderate to severe depression, even if for some of them they have no more than a placebo effect. It's estimated that for people with moderate to severe depression, if no treatment is given, 20 per cent will recover; if a placebo is given, 30 per cent will respond; and if an antidepressant is given, 50 per cent will respond. I imagine my pills giving him a surge of serotonin, his synapses now awash with the chemicals of happiness. At least resetting any chemical imbalance or deficit will give him the best possible chance of getting better. My scientific training warns me against it, but it's hard to ignore anecdotal evidence from personal experience – I have seen severely depressed and suicidal people improving beyond recognition after a few weeks of SSRIs. (As a junior hospital doctor I witnessed the same sort of miraculous recovery in severely depressed elderly patients after administering electroconvulsive therapy (ECT). I felt like a young Victor Frankenstein as I pressed the button, holding the electrode firmly against the patient's temple to induce a controlled seizure. It felt dark and brutal. No one really knows how it works, and there can be side effects, especially loss of memory – but for many, it can be life-saving.

There isn't much to choose between the different members of the SSRI family. The trials suggest they are all about as effective as each other. I choose antidepressants based on a range of things – for example, their side effects (sometimes it can be helpful, for instance, if they cause some sedation); any previous experiences, good or bad; and any other medications that the patient is on which might interact with them. But I chose Citalopram this time primarily because I know it well. I have grown used to it; it has become like a friend. I know its weaknesses and strengths, I trust it and it has not let me down over the years. It doesn't always work for every patient – sometimes we have to try a range of different antidepressants before we find one that suits – but most of the time it hits the spot.

I suppose I have a top twenty or so favourite medicines that I prescribe most of the time – my chosen 'drug squad'. For example, a couple of general-purpose antibiotics, antibiotics for specific problems, particular anti-hypertensives, a favourite oral contraceptive, Hormone Replacement Therapy, a familiar diuretic, steroids, skin creams, and a first-choice antidepressant. We've grown close over the years. Better to deal with a familiar squad of drugs than dabble with unknown ringers (however hard pharmaceutical representatives may try to squeeze a new one onto my team sheet). The downside of this intimacy is that it can be hard to adopt the latest unfamiliar recommended medication – it's like betraying a loved one. A doctor's love affair with a particular medicine often starts as a junior with a recommendation from a respected department head or consultant. Love blossoms with grateful patients' success stories, even as the doctor starts to appreciate the drug's weaknesses. We feel safe this way: we know intimately what we are giving our patients. Doctors know that drugs can be dangerous weapons and every doctor worries about harming patients by prescribing them. In the back of my mind is the Hippocratic maxim '*Premum non nocere*' or 'First do no harm'. In other words, before I reach for the electronic prescription pad, I always ask myself whether I might be making the patient worse off. Even as I sign a prescription for a simple anti-inflammatory, I have flashbacks to patients I have seen in hospital, with life threatening stomach bleeding from long term use of the same drug. And I'd better get the dose right. I once gave a young child ten times the normal dose of a powerful drug – I was so tired I put the decimal point in the wrong place. It was a toxic dose. She came back to hospital in a worse condition than when we sent her home a couple of days earlier. Fortunately, my default position was that anything that went wrong was probably my fault unless proven otherwise, and I checked the dose of drug I sent her home on. I came clean, told my boss and her parents, and thank God, we were able to make her better without any lasting damage. The parents were incredibly understanding. That's why I often look up doses of drugs, even ones in my drug squad, just to double-check – and particularly for children, where doses change progressively as they get older.

In my experience, used properly, antidepressants rarely cause serious problems; but of course there's no such thing as a free lunch and all medicines do have some side effects. The more common ones are things like nausea, difficulty sleeping (particularly not being able to get off to sleep) and sexual problems, especially a loss of desire for sex or finding it hard to have an orgasm. Apart from nausea, the SSRIs generally have fewer side effects than the older antidepressants (such as the tricyclics, which can cause drowsiness and a dry mouth, for example). They are also less dangerous in overdose; an important consideration in this group of patients.

Lots of patients are worried that they will be 'fobbed off' with anti-depressants, or that they will become addicted to them, turn into a Prozac zombie, or become suicidal. I really don't 'fob people off' with antidepressants. People accuse GPs of prescribing them like sweeties, but the decision is always complex and very rarely about a short-cut to end the consultation. The first thing to say is that if you have mild depression you almost certainly don't need antidepressants. In fact the latest evidence-based guidance for doctors from NICE says that in mild depression, the side effects may outweigh the benefits and you're more likely to do better with regular exercise (at least three times a week for forty-five minutes each time), reading self-help books or online programmes, or having some form of talking therapy such as counselling or cognitive behavioural therapy (CBT). For moderate depression, medication can be helpful combined with CBT. But most people with severe depression would probably benefit from antide-pressants. In every case, these are the sort of things I am weighing up: how antidepressants have certainly saved some of my patients' lives; the evidence that antidepressants can make people worse; the patient's wishes and beliefs (the placebo effect is powerful); the three-month wait before the patient will see a counsellor or CBT therapist; my estimate of the patient's risk of suicide (there are protocols for this); the severity of their depression (again, measurable); the recognised side effects; risks of overdose; any other medications the patient is taking; and so on.

SSRIs are not addictive in the true sense: they do not cause cravings or tolerance (where you need to take more and more of the drug to get the same effect). But there's no doubt you can get unpleasant, some-times serious, flu-like symptoms if you withdraw them too rapidly. So my advice to EK (as to everyone) was not to miss doses, and when the time comes to wean off them, do it very gradually under a doctor's guidance.

The main worry I have with EK is that when people first start on SSRIs their anxiety levels and suicidal thoughts can sometimes get worse before they get better. That is the main reason why I have brought him back today – the formal guidelines from NICE also recommend a check within one to two weeks of starting an SSRI. He was having suicidal thoughts last week, so I need to make sure things aren't worse now.

I already know that he is at high risk of killing himself. All the evidence suggests that being male, single, socially isolated, unemployed and depressed puts you in a fairly high risk bracket. Certain professions too, like doctors, vets and farmers, have higher rates of suicide than the general population. EK denies drinking much alcohol, so that's at least one risk factor that he doesn't have. Nor has he attempted suicide before – I asked him last week.

It can feel uncomfortable, even dangerous, talking to a depressed person about whether they have thought of killing themselves. Medical students often worry that it might tip someone over into actually acting out their suicidal thoughts. It crosses my mind too. But I try to reassure them, and myself, that there isn't any evidence to suggest that is the case. In fact most patients welcome the chance to share those thoughts with someone. Somehow it can make them seem less scary. I can also try to normalise them without downplaying them. It's not unusual, for example, for people to think about killing themselves, or to wonder about it, or to think that they might be better off dead. What I need to establish now is whether EK's thoughts have evolved into something more concrete since last week.

'Are you still having those thoughts about harming yourself?'

'Yes. I think I will be better off to die. I have nobody, and there's no point any more.'

'Have you made any plans to kill yourself?' I am asking the top of his head – he is still looking down, and thinking.

'Yes. I have many tablets. I will probably eat them all.'

'What sort of tablets do you have?'

'Codeine. Paracetamol.'

'How many have you collected?'

'Maybe three or four packets.'

'Of each?'

'Yes.'

Given that fewer paracetamol than that can cause liver damage and death, that concerns me. I have seen patients who have taken quite small amounts of paracetamol, more as a cry for help than a genuine suicide attempt, but by the time they come to the emergency department it's too late to give them an antidote. They can die a slow and unpleasant death from liver failure. And codeine in high doses can cause respiratory depression and death. The fact that EK has stored up medications, or says he has, makes me worried. Making active plans such as hoarding tablets or writing a note rings alarms bells. I have flashbacks of my crouching train lady.

'And how likely are you to take them, do you think? What, if anything, would stop you?'

Very often, people follow their description of suicidal thoughts with a rapid dismissal of the suggestion that they would act on them: 'Oh no, I could never do that. What about my children?' they say, or: 'No, I couldn't do that to my partner/dog/mistress.' It's an important part of my risk assessment.

'I worry that I might just do it one day. I have no one to talk with. No family is here. So why not?'

(ten minutes)

He sounds impulsive. He's worried that he might just do it – as if it's somehow out of his control. He's had many social and psychological stressors recently. He's in a high-risk demographic. Even his numbers match my hunch – his depression score on the PHQ-9 questionnaire is 22: 'severe'. He seems to be worse than last week. More than all this – he seems desperate. He reminds me of others I have seen, or heard about from colleagues, who have gone on to attempt or even commit suicide soon after seeing their GP. In the UK, suicide is the biggest killer of men under the age of forty-five – higher than road crashes, heart disease or cancer. One review of studies has estimated that 45 per cent of those dying by suicide saw their primary care physician in the month before their death. If someone really wants to kill themselves, there is little we can do to stop them – but I'll be damned if anyone kills themselves because I have not even tried to assess their suicidal risk properly.

'Look, I am worried about you. I think your depression has got a little worse since we last met. The pills won't start working for a week or more, and you are having some worrying thoughts about harming yourself now. I feel we should ask for advice now from the mental health specialists. Are you happy for me to do that?'

'Yes . . . OK.' He nods slowly.

I am aware that time is ticking by. I have now committed myself to trying to phone up my mental health colleagues to ask for their advice – hopefully to arrange some sort of urgent assessment with them. I take a deep breath – this could take a while. Can I afford to let the patient go home, and try to contact the psychiatric team after surgery? Or is he so much of a risk that I must ask him to stay here till I finish? Perhaps I should even phone them now, and risk adding another ten minutes or more onto my waiting time. Angry patients.

'Can I ring you after surgery? Do you have a mobile? It's just that it may take a little while for me to contact the team. I don't want to keep you here longer than you have to be.'

'Sure.' He gives me the number.

'Where will you go now?'

'To the café.'

'OK. I will call you in an hour or so; is that all right? Keep your phone on, will you? We'll get you seen to. Will you be OK until then, do you think?'

'Yes I think so.'

I'm happy he'll be in a public place. He has been thinking this way for a while and hasn't acted on it yet. He thinks he'll be OK. I will be phoning with help for him. So I judge that the risk that he will kill himself in the next hour or so is very small. Not zero, but small.

'OK, I will call you in an hour or so.'

'Thank you.'

He gets up to leave, with a furtive glance in my direction. I shadow him as he shuffles towards the door, my arms spread out around his shape, like a parent ushering a child along a tricky path.

Once he's gone, I reach for my big red book. I enter in his name and phone number, and my task: contact psych and phone patient. If it's in the red book it'll get done. I allow myself a few seconds to think about whether I've done the right thing. I then write the computer notes for our consultation; it helps me to gather my thoughts and pull together a coherent narrative, including a detailed record of my assessment of his suicidal risk. When I read it back to myself I think it just about justifies my actions, if anyone were to question them. It also helps me to prepare what I'm going to discuss with the psychiatrists on call in an hour or so.

The clock says I am now nearly twenty minutes late. Shit.

(15 minutes)

Chapter 6

Ms AW

(running eighteen minutes late)

Doctor view

Appointment time: 8.20
Name: Ms AW
Age: 45 years old
Occupation: Teacher
Past medical history:
  Migraine
  Back pain/sciatica
  Depression
  Allergic rhinitis
  Eczema
  Pneumonia
Medication:
  Citalopram (antidepressant)
Reminders:
  Smear overdue
  Measure weight (BMI >30)
Last consultation:
  For medical certificate (sick note) for
  back pain, two weeks' duration, ending
  today.
  Sciatica, seeing physio.

Patient view
*Ms AW is a divorced secondary school
teacher with two young children. Her
chronic back pain problems have flared up
again recently and she has had the last two
weeks off work. Her headmaster is putting
the pressure on her to come back – but the
job is so stressful at the moment, with a
school inspection looming, that she does
not feel ready to return. She really wants
another week off at least. She has also been
having terrible tummy pains over the last
few weeks, enough to make her feel sick.
They've even woken her up once. She is
concerned that this might be the sign of
something like appendicitis, or worse,
a bowel cancer.*

95

England are 210 for 5 in the Test Match. Not a great total, but Cook's still in and we have a reasonable middle-order. If we can just hold out until say, tea, then we're in with a chance. Consultation expert Roger Neighbour talks about the importance of what he calls 'housekeeping' for GPs – taking time to make sure you're OK and ready for the next patient. It could mean going to the toilet, a brief chat with the receptionists, checking my pigeon-hole for requests or queries from patients, or just taking a few slurps of coffee. I know some GPs who are into mindfulness meditation. For me, it's checking the cricket score online. I'm instantly at a sunny Lord's, the velvet green home of cricket (or, today, Eden Gardens in India), sipping an ale to the sound of polite applause and red leather on willow. It's the quickest way to clear my mind of the previous consultation, so that I can give the next patient my complete attention.

AW and I know each other quite well. I have accompanied her through several bouts of depression over the years and since I helped her through a nasty pneumonia about five years ago I think I've been her first-choice doctor in the practice. But she's not easy. She takes quite a bossy tone with me and is quite happy to criticise the other doctors, my colleagues. Although professionally I never collude with that kind of carping (in fact I often slap her down for it), inwardly I admit that it can give me a short-term ego boost. The trouble is that when someone finds it so easy to pillory others, you know it's only a matter of time before you become the object of their bile. We all understand that some patients gravitate towards certain doctors – they like this doctor's no-nonsense style, or that doctor's gentleness or humour, or they've built trust through sharing a significant illness together. We also know that patients often shop around – we can go in and out of fashion like tonsillectomies. We try not to take doctor-shopping personally; sometimes, to be honest, it's a relief when a patient moves on to someone else, able to offer a fresh pair of eyes on an old problem. What's good about my relationship with AW at the moment is that I know her well enough to be quite frank with her. I can be much more like the doctors I imagine of old; more direct, more paternalistic, even a bit rude. Like the Duke of Edinburgh. Sometimes, with some patients, that can be fun.

I'm now nearly twenty minutes late – I've nearly breached my own ideal limit for keeping patients waiting. I detest running late, although this is still some way off my 'personal worst' (nearly an hour, I'm afraid to say). I picture patients simmering in the waiting room, ready to explode at me when their turn finally comes round. It's happened before. I remember one blow-hard who bellowed at me in front of an open-mouthed waiting room, moaning that he had been kept waiting for half an hour, that it was unacceptable, that I was unprofessional, and that he was a very busy man. I remember trembling, partly from shock, partly from indignation. I had just been dealing with a patient who was having a heart attack. That takes a little longer than ten minutes. Because of patient confidentiality, I couldn't tell him what I had been tackling in the previous consultation, so I just had to apologise, explain that it was a complicated case, and take his public tantrum on the chin. That experience, and a few others like it, lurks at the back of my mind whenever I step over my self-imposed twenty-minute-wait limit.

I take a deep breath, edge out to the waiting room and call AW's name. She heaves herself up, as if trying to overcome some giant magnetic force sucking her back down to the brown plastic banquette. I know she has an attractive face, a mischievous smile even, when she's in a good mood. But today it's an ugly pain-face. Her eyes are almost shut as she shambles slowly towards me, whimpering with every lurch.

'I'm so sorry to keep you waiting,' I say. I mean it.

She is concentrating so hard on showing me her pain that she ignores my apology completely. No eye contact at all. It's a relief in one way – she doesn't mind that she's been kept waiting. But I am now preparing for a high-stakes meeting; she's telling me that this level of discomfort is serious, not something to be taken lightly, not for 'fobbing off'. I am not denying her pain – but I think I can usually tell when familiar patients deliberately turn up the pain volume a few notches for my benefit. It's her way of telling me this really hurts.

'That looks painful,' I say, hoping that acknowledging her performance might allow her to tone it down a bit.

'Oh, it's terrible,' she sighs, as she slumps into the chair.

'How on earth are you managing?' I ask.

'Not at all well. I think it's much worse.'

97

'In what way is it worse?'

'The pain is just really getting me down now . . . sometimes I don't know what to do with myself.'

I listen carefully to her symptoms and how they are affecting her. I know back pain is deeply unpleasant, like a gnawing toothache in the spine. Sciatica is any sort of pain caused by irritation or compression of the sciatic nerve. The sciatic nerve is the longest nerve in the body and it travels from the lower spine, through the buttocks and down the legs to the feet. When the nerve is squashed or irritated – usually by a bulging (or 'slipped' – not an accurate term really) disc as it emerges from the lower spine – it can cause pain, numbness or tingling anywhere from the buttocks down one of your legs to your toes on that side. GPs see lots of back pain, with or without sciatica; it affects around one-third of the adult UK population each year and out of these patients around 20 per cent will go to a GP for consultation (that's around 2.6 million people each year).

AW has a long history of back pain and sciatica – it has in effect become a chronic, long-term condition for her. Every now and then she gets a flare-up, and needs time off work. When back pain is at its worst, it would be very hard, if not impossible, for her to teach a class effectively. Not necessarily because her back pain interferes mechanically with the physical aspects of her job – but because when you have pain gnawing away at your nerve like a dogged rodent, it's impossible to do much else at all.

It fascinates me how pain is so closely interwoven with the mind. Pain can make you frustrated, stressed, frightened, depressed – all of which, we know, can affect how you perceive pain and how you use your body, perhaps trying to protect a painful region. That can lead to a downward spiral of worsening pain, unhelpful emotions and further disability. The Cartesian view of physical pain – that it's somehow separate from the mind – seems so obviously misguided to me. In fact we know that tackling the psychological aspects is often the key to helping people with chronic pain. The stress of AW's job right now may well be an important factor in all of this. But I have to tread very carefully before I step into that tiger country.

I have had a peculiar personal experience of the power of the mind over pain. When I was working in an emergency department during my training (GPs spend at least three years of their training in hospital posts) I had a minor operation on my penis. It was an abnormal patch of skin which needed a biopsy – it later turned out to be nothing serious. But while I was working on my night shift in the emergency department, the stitches broke and the wound started to bleed quite heavily. I weighed up my options. I was surrounded by professionals who could have easily stitched it up again for me – but I knew them all as friends or work colleagues. Too embarrassing. Or I could stitch it up myself. A bit weird. For me, weird wins over embarrassing every time. (Although here I am, writing about it.) So I went to the shelf for some fine suture, the sharpest needle I could find, tweezers and some swabs. I decided not to take any local anaesthetic – sometimes the injection for the local anaesthetic is more painful than just getting on with the stitching. I snuck off to my on-call room in a rare quiet moment, and started to prepare the haemorrhaging organ by swabbing and cleaning it. What was strange was that I put three separate stitches into the wound without feeling any real pain. I think I was so focused on doing a good job that my mind was too occupied to entertain any fear. And there's something about being in control, too, which reduces the fear factor, and therefore the pain. It's a bit like being in the driving seat, rather than cowering in the back seat entirely dependent on someone else's judgement and skill. In a similar way, patients feel much better when they understand their pain and feel they have at least some control over it.

'I am going to need another certificate. The old one runs out today.'

'OK, that's no problem. What do you think – another week?' I reach for the pad of sick notes in my drawer. This is not normally such a reflex action. But I know her well, I'm keen to catch up on some time if I can – and here is a gift. A short form, a stamp and a signature. Patient happy, doctor happy.

In the UK patients can sign themselves off sick for up to seven calendar days. After that, they have to come to me. I resent having to juggle the conflicting roles of work-fitness policeman and patient advocate. I went in to this career to help patients, to support them. Now here I am, forced to make a judgement about my patient's fitness for work – but I don't have the time or the training to make a proper occupational assessment (there are doctors who specialise in that sort of thing). Nor is it really possible for me to make an objective judgement about a patient's level of pain, or how it might affect their work role. I can ask her how painful it is on a scale of 1 to 10, or ask her to walk from one side of my room to the other, even examine the range of movement in her joints and check her nervous system. If someone says they are stressed and anxious, I can only judge the impact of their symptoms on their work by asking them. But nearly all of those measurements are subjective and open to exaggeration by a patient. Sometimes I do get the sense that they are swinging the lead, in which case we have a frank discussion, and I might suggest limited work duties or even refuse to sign a certificate. But it's not an exact science, it's more of a hunch. It also completely changes the dynamic of the doctor–patient relationship – it becomes more adversarial than supportive, and the hard-won trust at the heart of general practice can crumble away in the flourish of a pen. Better for an expert independent assessor, taking account of the GP's knowledge of the patient over the years, to make those kind of judgements. In the UK that only happens after a certain period of time, or when a patient makes a claim for benefits.

'Yes, please. Maybe a week or two?'

'Well, let's say a week for now, and we can always reassess things in a week's time if needed. What did we put last time – just back pain and sciatica?'

'Yes, I think so.'

I scribble the note, rip the page out, and hand it over to her.

(*three minutes*)

The research suggests that most back pain (up to 90 per cent of cases) will get better within six weeks, no matter what you do. The idea that it might take up to six weeks before things improve can be depressing news for patients, but it can also be a useful yardstick when it comes to making decisions about what to do. I can test for sciatic nerve involvement when I examine a patient: when the patient raises their straight leg up off the couch, they get sciatic pain as the nerve is stretched. I check for any effects on the peripheral nervous system in their legs too: the tone of muscle groups in the leg (are the muscles relaxed or stiff?), their power (any major weakness can be a sign of nerve damage), how responsive they are to sensation (usually tested with a wisp of cotton wool, comparing different areas supplied by specific nerves), and the reflexes (gently tapping the tendon at the front of the knee, or at the back of the ankle. Generally, decreased reflexes indicate a problem with the peripheral nerves, and lively or exaggerated reflexes, like a Karate kick, a problem with the central nervous system).

People often expect an X-ray or an MRI scan, but for the vast majority of back pain cases, those investigations don't tell us much and, more importantly, even if they show up a bulging disc, don't usually alter the clinical management at that stage. They can also expose people to an unnecessary dose of radiation: an X-ray of the lower spine gives you roughly the same radiation dose as about fifty chest X-rays (the dose needs to be higher to penetrate the denser bones in your vertebrae). So, last time, I gave her the usual evidence-based advice: keep moving, stay as active as possible, and try simple painkillers like paracetamol or ibuprofen. I also referred her to a private physiotherapist – she has the insurance, and the NHS waiting time to see a physio at the moment in my area is about six weeks at least. Not ideal.

What I must do today though is check that her back pain doesn't have any worrying features. I'm not deeply concerned but I would expect it to be getting a bit better after two weeks. Rushing through my mind are cauda equina syndrome, an infection of the spine, a spinal fracture, or cancer. Cauda equina syndrome is a rare but serious condition that can cause sciatica. The cauda equina (the Latin for horse's tail) is the bundle of nerves that lead out from the end of the spinal cord – if these are compressed and damaged it can eventually lead to paralysis if left untreated. The warning signs of cauda equina syndrome are suddenly losing control of your bladder or bowels, tingling or numbness in the 'saddle area' (round the anus and between the upper inner thighs), or weakness in the leg or foot. Spinal fractures normally cause pain that comes on suddenly, caused by trauma such as a traffic accident or a fall – there's nothing like that here. I think about cancer or infection if someone has a history of cancer (it might have spread to the spine), if they're over fifty or under twenty, if they have a fever or unexplained weight loss, or if they get constant pain, waking them at night. As with many cancer sufferers, my father's kidney cancer first showed itself as back pain and weight loss. The undiagnosed primary cancer in his kidney had spread to the spine. He had the non-deliberate weight loss and lack of appetite that often accompanies advanced cancer (so-called cachexia). When I look back, I should have spotted the signs earlier than I did – my excuse is that Dad was stoical, he downplayed it extremely persuasively, and it was hard for me to question his authority as my father and an experienced senior doctor. Doctors often ignore their symptoms for too long. He died only a few months later.

'Have you got any weakness in the leg?'

'Mmm. Maybe a little; it doesn't feel quite as strong as usual.'

A little weakness sometimes goes with sciatica. She's having to think about it hard – I don't sense a big deterioration there.

'Any problems with water works, or opening your bowels?'

'No, that's OK. But I am getting these tummy pains that I really need to talk to you about.'

'OK, we'll come back to that.' My heart sinks; another problem I must tackle. Another four or five minutes, minimum.

'Any numbness or tingling around the bottom area?'

'No.'

So I'm happy now that there are no alarm signs here; her back pain and sciatica are painful but stable. The advice hasn't changed.

'Can you manage for now on the same painkillers?'

'Yes, I think so. I know it will just take some time to settle, and the physio is helping.'

Now for the 'tummy pain'.

(*six minutes*)

'OK, so you mentioned some pain in your tummy. Tell me more about that.'

Most abdominal pain we see in general practice is temporary and non-serious. Transient and trivial. Gastroenteritis, constipation, a bit of wind – that sort of thing. I'm hoping it'll be that, but I have to assess it properly each time – occasionally it will be something more serious like appendicitis, bowel obstruction, or an ulcer. The potential list is long. People often worry that abdominal pain could mean cancer – that is not high on my list, because it very rarely does.

'Well, for the last two weeks or so, I suppose. But it's got worse. It makes me feel sick.'

'Are you actually sick?' Vomiting could mean anything from gastro-enteritis – but that rarely lasts more than a few days – to serious bowel obstruction (a blockage), which usually goes with constipation and colicky pains.

'No, I just feel like I might be sick.'

'And whereabouts do you get it?'

'It's over here mostly.' She waves towards the upper part of her abdomen – not precisely, more of a rough indication of a region.

The location of any pain is probably my number one diagnostic clue. I suppose that's why I spent so long at medical school with my hands inside a corpse. At the time, it felt pointless and brutal, if a little thrilling at eighteen years old. A group of five of us spent hours each day for two years slowly picking apart a dead body, generously donated by someone who wanted to help medical science. We all had enormous admiration and gratitude for those people and their relatives. We were very clear that if there was any sense of disrespect-ful behaviour, we would have been severely reprimanded or thrown off the course. But I always felt that 'medical science' was a very loose description of what we were doing. We'd hold an instruction manual in one hand, and a scalpel in the other, occasionally pointing out an organ or a nerve or a blood vessel that we thought we'd spotted. It was hopeless. 'Isn't that the pancreas?' someone would ask. 'Or is it the stomach?' 'No, I don't think so, it's just a bit of fat, or maybe omentum?' The omentum is a large apron-like lining that hangs down from the stomach.

103

The bodies were preserved in formalin, which made accurate dissection and identification of body parts very tricky, even in expert hands. But in the hands of a bunch of hungover teenagers, it was like a team of toddlers trying to fillet a fish with a knife and fork. When it came to learning anatomy of the limbs, we would have to saw an arm off, or a leg, to make it easier to manipulate and dissect. Every morning we'd come in and gather round a large tub of formalin with ten or so arms floating around in it. You'd identify yours by checking the name tag tied to a finger or a toe – if it wasn't yours, you'd return it with a splash and try another one. It was like some ghoulish fairground hook-the-duck game.

We certainly learned from those bodies. We were tested fully and regularly. But personally, I learned most of my anatomy from beautifully drawn textbooks. I'm glad to say that, these days, students learn from professionally dissected body specimens and three-dimensional computer images, which are great for understanding all the complex layers and relations of the human form. The link between the pure anatomy and the real clinical work of a doctor is now made much more apparent. But without any obvious relevance, I found anatomy deadly boring, and failed both my first and second years' exams at the first attempt. It's only now, after years of clinical work, that I would really find anatomy dissection useful, fascinating even.

But looking back there was great value in those hands-on dissection days, and my time assisting in surgical operations as a junior hospital doctor. I can now bring to mind an idealised visceral landscape, a fairly accurate facsimile of this lady's insides. I suppose it's a bit like having slightly out-of-focus X-ray vision. We are taught to think of the abdomen divided up into zones. Imagine a giant game of noughts and crosses drawn on it. When we are describing where pain is, we think and talk in terms of right upper quadrant (RUQ), left upper quadrant (LUQ), the epigastrium (central upper abdomen), right iliac fossa (the lower right side), left iliac fossa (left lower side), and suprapubic (just above the pubic bone) and central regions (right in the middle).

Different causes of abdominal pain tend to cause pain in particular areas, related to the position of the main organs. For some causes, the link between location of pain and the position of the underlying culprit is very close. For example, pain in the right iliac fossa is highly predictive of appendicitis. The appendix is a finger-like pouch that comes off the large bowel, usually in the lower right side of your abdomen (the right iliac fossa). In appendicitis the appendix gets inflamed – swollen and painful. Typically the pain starts in the very centre of the abdomen, and then moves down to focus (or 'localise' to use the medical parlance) in the right iliac fossa. But as with everything in medicine, it doesn't always behave according to this textbook description – in rare cases, some people even have their appendix on the left side. In pregnant women, the swollen womb pushes the appendix high up under the ribs on the right side – I have seen a case of appendicitis in a pregnant woman which presented as pain in the right upper quadrant. Not typical at all.

Epigastric pain, on the other hand (high up in the middle of the abdomen), is often associated with stomach problems (ulcers), pancreatitis or oesophagitis – the stomach, the pancreas and the oesophagus (or gullet; the food pipe) are all in that region. But frequently the location of the pain is rather generalised, or isn't a terribly helpful predictor of the underlying cause. Unfortunately, lots of things can cause rather generalised pain – including gastroenteritis (very common), irritable bowel syndrome (also common), excess wind, and the one you don't want me to miss: generalised peritonitis (inflammation of the peritoneum, the abdominal lining, which is often caused by something serious like a burst appendix or perforated bowel).

AW is pointing roughly to an area covering the epigastrium, and the right upper quadrant. In other words, the upper central and right side of her abdomen, from her perspective (in anatomy we always describe things from the perspective of the patient – the patient's right side, not the right side as I look at it). In my mind I am taking a miniature helicopter ride, flying over this bit of her insides. High up under her ribs on her right side is the liver – a giant glistening red-brown wedge. Nestling underneath it is her gall-bladder, like a little gourd, and its tubes or ducts which carry the bile into the small bowel. I have spent many hours directing an internal camera at this part of patients' insides, so that my surgeon boss could get at the gall-bladder underneath. I have handled many gall-bladders and bowels – I imagine what hers might feel like between my fingers. Then there's the small intestine, loops of shiny grey tubing – including the duodenum, the first bit that leads out from the stomach. As I hover towards her midline, here is the stomach, like the floppy bag of a set of bagpipes; the oesophagus is the pipe sprouting upwards from it, through a hole in the sheet-like diaphragm which divides the chest from the abdomen. Hiding behind her stomach is the pancreas, controller of sugar and digestive-juice maker, like a giant yellowy tongue, sticking out horizontally across her abdomen.

There are lots of things that can go wrong with all these bits. That's what we learned in pathology (in anatomy we studied the normal, and in pathology we studied the abnormal), and from seeing the range of clinical cases during our training. As a GP, I'm thinking about common things first – as the saying goes 'common things happen commonly'. Medical students, who know much more than I do about all the pathological fascinomas (interesting or unusual cases/diagnoses), often come up with the rarest diagnosis imaginable as their best bet because they haven't yet had the clinical experience to work out a realistic order of likelihood. A keen and knowledgeable student, for example, might suggest Budd-Chiari syndrome (a rare condition caused by a blockage of veins in the liver) as the number one diagnosis rather than the much more likely pain from the gall-bladder.

I remember being asked, on day one of our training on the wards, for the possible causes of a cough. Most people off the street would be able to give you a few sensible suggestions – a viral infection like influenza, asthma, pneumonia. But after two years of learning theory from textbooks and lectures, none of us could think of anything more likely than tuberculosis and pulmonary embolism (a blood clot on the lungs). I think that is also a trap that patients can fall into when they look up their symptoms on the internet. They type in 'pain in the right upper abdomen', and up pops a list as long as your small intestine (about seven metres by the way) including rarities like subphrenic abscess (a collection of pus under the diaphragm), renal cancer, and Budd-Chiari syndrome. It must be hard to make sense of all the possibilities without years of clinical experience, and without the benefit of the focused and objective questioning that doctors are taught to use to sift the 'could be serious' from the 'probably isn't'. I've got to be aware of the unusual, of course, but in first-opinion medicine I won't do the patient any favours by leaping, House-like, for the diagnosis which is as rare as rocking horse shit, as my tutor used to say.

My immediate thoughts are leaning towards the commoner causes of right upper quadrant pain, like inflammation of the gall bladder (cholecystitis) or biliary colic (spasm of the bile ducts), and I'm not excluding the more epigastric problems like ulcers, gastritis, oesophagitis, or even pancreatitis. That's because of where her pain is, and what I know about the sort of people who are more likely to get those problems.

Stomach ulcers, for instance, are often triggered by taking non-steroidal anti-inflammatories like ibuprofen (she's been taking those for her back pain over the last few weeks). Surgeons used to use the adage 'fair, fat, fertile, female and forty' as a mnemonic for those most likely to develop gall-stones. We now know that's only part of the story, but it's true that gallstones are more common in women, with increasing age, and in woman taking oral contraceptives. Most people with gall-stones don't have any symptoms at all – only about 10–25 per cent will ever get any problems with them. The main risk is what is known as biliary colic – an intermittent pain caused by a gall-stone getting stuck in the duct that carries bile from the gall-bladder to the bowel.

If knowing the location of the pain is the number one clue, then knowing its nature – what the pain is like – is probably number two.

'And how would you describe the pain? Is it sharp and stabbing, or more of a dull ache?'

'It's more of a dull ache I suppose, but very painful.'

'And does it come and go, or is it there all the time?'

Doctors have different words to describe the different types of pain you can feel in the abdomen. Very broadly, pains may be sharp or stabbing, crampy, colicky or a general dull ache. Patients don't always use these shorthand terms of course – or if they do, they don't mean what I mean by them. So it's really important for me to understand exactly what the patient is trying to describe.

Constant dull or aching abdominal pain is usually caused by the stretching or swelling of the wall of a hollow organ, or when the capsules that cover solid organs like the liver are stretched, say from inflammation.

Colicky pain or crampy pains, on the other hand, gradually become worse, then ease off again. This may happen repeatedly, coming and going in waves of pain. Imagine wringing a wet towel tightly, and then relaxing it. This sort of colicky pain is usually associated with contractions of a tubular or hollow structure surrounded by smooth muscle – so, typically, the bowel itself or other tubes such as those that carry urine from the kidneys to the bladder (the ureters; hence ureteric colic) or the gall-bladder or the ducts from the gall-bladder (hence biliary colic). The pain comes in waves because the smooth muscle that lines these tubes contracts and relaxes rhythmically to help the contents – for example, faeces, urine, bile – move along the tube's length. When there's a blockage like a bowel tumour or hard stools or a kidney stone, the muscles start working harder to try to dislodge the problem and that's what is often so painful. Just to confuse the issue, biliary colic is actually a constant dull aching pain as the gall-bladder is stretched (because the duct leading from it is blocked by a stone). Then, when the gall-bladder contracts against the obstruction, the stretch of the gall-bladder wall is suddenly intensified, producing a crescendo of pain in addition to the constant dull ache already present.

People rarely come in describing their pain as it is described in the textbooks. I'd fall off my chair if AW came in giving a textbook description of biliary colic: 'I have been getting constant intense pains in my right upper quadrant, radiating through to my scapula (shoulder blade). It lasts a few minutes, occasionally longer, and can be colicky in nature. I've noticed that it's worse when I eat fatty foods, and I can sometimes feel sick with it.' So it's my job to recognise typical elements in the story, to listen out for strong clues, to ask specifically about key features if I suspect a particular problem, to exclude other possibilities (especially red flags), and to piece together a likely picture from all the bits: the patient's risk factors, the symptoms they describe, what makes it better or worse, and the examination findings.

'It comes for about ten or fifteen minutes. Then it settles down. It's really bad when it comes though.'

'What score would you give it if zero was no pain and ten was the worst pain you've ever had?'

'Oh, eight or nine at least.'

It's a crude scale, but it can help when patients are struggling with their descriptive language – it's hard for me to grasp fully what someone means by 'really bad' or 'terrible'.

'And have you noticed if anything makes it better or worse?'

'It's worse after I eat sometimes.'

'Does any particular food trigger it?'

I'm thinking of fatty foods here – a typical feature of biliary colic because the gall-bladder wants to contract to release bile into the bowel to help with digestion of fatty foods. And that makes the pain worse. If it was the gnawing pain of a duodenal ulcer, it might be relieved by eating food, and ulcer pain is typically worse at night. So it doesn't sound like an ulcer.

'Not that I've noticed.'

(*nine minutes*)

Oh well. You rarely get the perfect pattern. These are all just pointers. On the other hand, there may well be a close link with fatty foods – it's just that she hasn't noticed that it's much worse after cheese on toast or a big slice of cake.

'And what can you do to make it better?' Anything help?'

'Paracetamol sometimes helps a bit.'

If she had an ulcer, gastritits or oesophagitis, she might be more likely to say 'Rennie's' or 'Gaviscon' – the anti-acid medications that you can buy off the shelf. Painkillers are often more helpful with biliary colic.

I'm also interested in whether the pain seems to be travelling (radiating) in a certain direction. For example, biliary colic sometimes radiates through to the shoulder blade – but she doesn't have that symptom. I quickly ask questions designed to pick up on the worrying red flags we are trained to look for in upper abdominal pain. I sometimes forgot to ask about key red flags when I was a trainee; even missing one or two basic questions could spell failure in the clinical GP exam.

'No weight loss or blood in your stools? No change in your bowel habits? No trouble swallowing?' (These would make me worry about cancer.)

'No.'

'OK, thanks. Can I have a quick feel of your tummy in that case?'

'Yes, of course.'

'Come up and lie down on the couch here . . .' I pull down some protective paper for the couch from the giant toilet-roll holder at the head end of my couch. 'There you go.'

She bends down in painful slow motion to try to undo her laces.

'Don't bother to take your shoes off . . . just jump up.'

I have to stop myself from getting frustrated and short with people at this point. There's often so much fiddling about with clothes and shoes, and wondering which way to lie, that I can lose several minutes just getting someone into the position we are taught to get them in for an abdominal examination: lying flat, abdomen exposed (ideally from 'nipples to knees', but realistically, from bottom of ribcage to top of loosened trousers or skirt). It can feel like I'm waiting in a pointless traffic jam, late for a job interview. It's not the patient's fault of course – the system provides the time pressure, and I just need to be very clear with my instructions. And tolerant. I count to ten.

I'm still information-gathering. I have 'taken the patient's history', focusing on the questions relating to upper abdominal pains, and adapted to the answers she has given. I've tried to ask her open questions to let her tell her own story – but frankly I've not done a great job there. So far I have asked lots of closed questions, like a rapid-fire machine gun. Maybe while I am examining her, I could give her a little space to tell me more about what she thinks might be the problem. It's always helpful to know that (not because I have no idea, just because I can then address what's going on in her mind).

'OK.' I rub my hands to warm them a bit. An empathetic touch, literally, which we're taught in training.

'So what do you make of these pains? Have you had any thoughts about what it might be?'

'I've no idea. You're the doctor.' Unnecessarily snappy, I think. But that may be because she's actually worried about something, and too embarrassed to say.

'Yes, I know – and I have my own thoughts – but sometimes people wonder if it might be this or that, and it helps me to know what you're thinking about.'

'No, I don't have any thoughts about it at all.'

'OK.' I smile. I have tried my best. 'I'm just going to press softly to start with – OK?'

We're taught a system for examining the abdomen. As for every examination, it should start with inspection – a general look at her whole body, and then more focused on the face and mouth and hands. At least, that is what I would expect students to do in their final exams. You can find important clues – obvious ones like extreme weight loss or jaundice (yellowing of the skin or the whites of the eyes, often signifying a problem with the liver), or more subtle ones like spider naevi (spidery veins over the upper body, which can also point to liver problems, or excess alcohol), Dupuytren's contracture (a thickening of the palms of the hand which can cause 'clawing' of the fingers, sometimes linked to diabetes or alcoholic excess, but that can also run in families – British prime minister Margaret Thatcher famously had it) or mouth ulcers (the gut starts at the lips and ends at the anal margin).

But today I don't have time to do a final grade examination – this is a rapid assessment. It's not about cutting corners, it's about being efficient; what we call a focused examination. It becomes easier with practice. If there were any worrying features, I'd revert to the full final version of the physical examination. I do have a look at the whites of her eyes to check for jaundice though, and at her face, checking for any obvious 'spiders'.

Feeling, or palpating, the abdomen should follow a system covering all the main areas. I start softly, like gently kneading dough, and watch the patient's facial expressions closely. You fail your medical exams if you don't notice that you're hurting the patient (because, for example, you have your nose pointing at their tummy button, not their face). As I press each region, I am imagining the structures within. As I start to feel more deeply the next time round, my fingers are scanning for the main organs – clockwise from the right upper quadrant, its liver, transverse colon, stomach, pancreas, spleen, descending colon, bladder – and checking for any discomfort or 'tenderness' on palpation. Tenderness usually indicates some inflammation – possibly infection. Someone with peritonism (inflammation of the inner abdominal lining – the peritoneum), say from a burst appendix, will usually be so tender that they hold their abdomen rigid like a plank. They often exhibit what we call 'guarding' when you try to press on the abdomen – tensing of the abdominal wall muscles to guard inflamed organs within the abdomen from the pain of pressure – the French call it '*défense musculaire*'. Another classic test of peritonism is to press deeply, gently and slowly in one spot – say over the right iliac fossa if I suspect appendicitis – and then suddenly to release the pressure by lifting my hand away rapidly. Typically, it's not as painful when I'm pressing down slowly on the abdomen as it is when I suddenly release the pressure – the peritoneum is suddenly stretched or aggravated and the patient pretty much jumps off the couch. Testing for rebound tenderness has gone out of fashion in recent years – apart from it being pretty close to a form of torture, some have questioned how useful it is over and above the other signs and symptoms of peritonism.

From the history, I admit I would have at least liked to find some tenderness over the right upper quadrant to bolster my gall-bladder theory. Or perhaps some epigastric discomfort to lead me in a more oesophageal or gastric direction. But nothing. I feel for both kidneys, using both hands – one hand pushes up from the back, and the other tries to feel at the front. Kidneys are much more 'round the back' than you might think – if you had to draw where they were on someone with a marker pen, you'd draw the kidneys on the back, just to either side of the spine, tucked under the lower edge of the ribcage. And you can't normally feel a left kidney, except in very thin people. You can sometimes feel the lower end of the right kidney. But if there's a mass, say a tumour, they can become enlarged so that you can feel them more easily. Everything normal in AW.

I feel for her liver now – or at least its lower edge, which sometimes pokes out from under the lower margin of the ribcage on the right-hand side. I am feeling for the liver edge with the flat of my hand, my fingers parallel to the lowest rib. As I do this, I ask AW to breathe in and out as I try to coordinate her breaths with a gentle upward movement of my fingertips. This takes practice. But once you have felt a liver edge it becomes second nature; I imagine it's rather like milking a cow to a dairy maid. An enlarged liver – say more than two to three fingers' width below the lower rib – could be a sign of liver pathology. As a student I was once caught out by a hugely enlarged liver – extending right down from the right lower ribs to the lower abdomen. I started feeling for an 'edge' high up near the ribs where it normally is. Nothing to feel, so I said it was normal. But of course the edge of this massively swollen liver (in this case from cirrhosis) was much lower down. The lesson – as my consultant helpfully pointed out – was to feel for a liver edge low down if you can't obviously feel one high up. As a student, it's easy to start thinking in terms of 'livers' and 'edges' rather than people.

High up in the left side of your abdomen, tucked under your ribcage near your back, is the spleen. The spleen is part of the lymphatic system – it maintains healthy red and white blood cells and platelets; platelets help your blood clot. It also filters blood, removing abnormal blood cells from the bloodstream. A normal-sized spleen is about the size of a fist and is usually impossible to feel. In fact, the trouble with the spleen is that even when it's enlarged it's often impossible to feel. The experts at feeling spleens are the haematologists (the blood specialists), whose patients frequently have enlarged spleens from conditions like leukaemia or lymphoma (cancers of the blood or lymphatic system). Because it is so challenging to feel a spleen, normal or abnormal, my examination in that quadrant is often a little rudimentary, dismissive even. But if for any reason I suspect a spleen might be enlarged (and there are many causes, including infections like glandular fever, or inflammatory conditions like rheumatoid arthritis) I will make a special effort to hunt for it.

If there's any doubt about enlarged livers or spleens, I can 'percuss' over them – tap across them using my fingertip like a mini hammer, usually against a finger of my opposite hand lying on the organ in question. This is just the same as plumbers or builders tapping on walls to see if they are hollow or solid. If you move your tapping finger across an organ, when the sound changes from a dull thud (solid organ) to a more resonant tap (hollow abdominal cavity or bowel) you have located the edge of a solid organ. I take pride in my percussion skills – I probably linger a little on this bit. When the rhythm and weight of each tap is just right, my fingers become like midget drums, beating out the sounds of shapes.

As every medical student knows, an abdominal examination is not complete without a rectal examination and examination of the external genitalia, the lymph nodes in the groin, and the hernial orifices (the holes in the abdominal muscles through which bits of bowel can sometimes push through causing a hernia). And, of course, women have all sorts of important bits in the lower abdomen and pelvis which can complicate the abdominal examination considerably. But today, for Ms AW, I decide to spare her, and me, any meaningful inspection of those bits because I judge that it is most unlikely that her upper abdominal symptoms have anything to do with the lower parts of her abdomen.

I have a quick listen to her abdomen with my stethoscope. I'm listening for bowel sounds – just like the sounds you sometimes hear 'out loud' when your stomach's making grumbling noises when you're hungry. The intestines are hollow, so bowel sounds echo through the abdomen like the sound of water in drains. It's normal to hear bowel sounds – it just means the intestine is working. When the bowel is very active, say with diarrhoea, the bowel sounds become noisier and more frequent. If there are no bowel sounds to hear, the intestines are inactive – this could signal a condition called ileus where the bowel stops its normal rhythmic muscle contractions (that can happen after some types of bowel surgery, for example). If there's a mechanical blockage in the bowel – say from a tumour, or old scar tissue, or a section of twisted bowel – you can often hear very high-pitched tinkling bowel sounds, like tiny droplets of water dripping down from the ceiling of a drain to the water below. It all sounds normal in Ms AW.

This is pretty typical general practice. No clear diagnosis yet, but some possibilities more likely than others. My goal is to sort out a sensible management plan, including any investigations, and to cover any worst-case scenarios. Unlike hospital doctors, we can easily ask patients to come back to take another look in a few days' or weeks' time.

(***eleven minutes***)

'OK, thanks. That's all done. Get yourself dressed and come and sit down and we'll talk about it.'

As I stand at my little basin scrubbing my hands with my back to her, gathering my thoughts, she kicks things off.

'What did you find then?'

'Well, examining you, everything seems OK – certainly nothing to worry about. But I think from your symptoms that this could be down to gall-stones.' I watch her reaction carefully to see how this is going down.

'Mmm. Well, no one ever told me I have gall-stones. Could it be my appendix?'

Earlier she told me she didn't have any thoughts at all about what this could be. Still, now it's out in the open we can tackle it head on.

'No, I don't think so. You certainly don't have the typical symptoms or signs of appendicitis. It's much more likely – with pains coming and going high up here (I point to my right upper quadrant) – that it's your gall-bladder. Anyway, what I think would be useful would be to get an ultrasound scan of your abdomen to see if you have gall-stones as a first step. And we'll organise some blood tests too.' Ultrasound scans are great for spotting gall-stones. And as for blood tests, I'm thinking particularly of tests for liver function, and pancreatitis, as well as a general check of her full blood count. I'll probably get a urine sample too, to exclude a urine infection.

'Can you manage the pain while we do that? It may take a week or so . . .'

'Well, paracetamol isn't helping much. Can't you give me something stronger?'

'I can give you a more powerful painkiller – a mix of paracetamol and codeine. It can make you a bit constipated though. You might need to take a laxative at the same time.'

'Well, I don't want to get constipated, do I?'

'No. Sorry – I sometimes cause more problems than I solve with my medicines, don't I? I'll give you some laxatives. And of course, don't take the painkillers as well as your paracetamol – these new ones already have paracetamol in them. Are you happy with that plan?'

'Yes – and when do I come back to see you again, because you're hardly ever here?'

'I know. I'm a part-timer. Hopeless.' She mentions this quite a lot, and I do feel bad that it's not easier for people like her to see me regularly. Even though I've explained before that I teach medical students and trainee GPs for the rest of the week, she likes to have a little dig whenever she can.

'Well, make an appointment to see me as soon as you can after the ultrasound scan. Obviously if the pain gets worse before then, you must see any doctor here urgently. If it gets really uncomfortable, the emergency department at the hospital is probably the best place. Is that OK?'

I don't really have time – but the computer is bullying me to measure her weight and remind her about her cervical smear. I'm late already; just do it . . .

'Before you go, it's been a while since we measured your weight – can you quickly jump on the scales for me?'

She snails over to the scales and eventually the pointer just about settles on 103 kg. That's 3 kg more than two years ago, but I don't want to get into discussions about weight loss right now – we've talked about it many times before; apart from anything else, it could really help her back pain problems. I enter her weight, and the computer calculates her BMI. More points.

'And will you organise your smear with the nurse – I think that's overdue now, isn't it?'

'Yes, OK.'

The comforting whirr of the printer signals the end of the consultation. I hand over the prescription and start writing up my records. I make a note of my differential diagnoses, with gall-stones at the top of the list, and the plan. I'm not sure what the diagnosis is yet; but I have some ideas and now I need to test them out with some investigations, and time. I also enter a reminder of what might be the next steps if she comes back and things haven't improved or become any clearer after the scan. It's partly for me, but partly for any colleagues who might see her next. 'If not settling consider bloods and/or referral for endoscopy.'

(*13 minutes*)

Chapter 7

Mrs JI

*(**running twenty-two minutes late**)*

Doctor view

Appointment time: 8.30
Name: Mrs JI
Age: 55 years old
Occupation: Housewife
Past medical history:
   Asthma
   Hysterectomy
   Depression
   Cholecystectomy (gall-bladder removal)
   Excision of skin tag on neck
   Hypertension (high blood pressure)
   Diabetes
Medication:
   Salbutamol inhaler for asthma
   Beclometasone inhaler for asthma
   Metformin for diabetes
   ACE inhibitor for blood pressure
   HRT (Hormone Replacement Therapy)
Reminders:
   Asthma annual review overdue
   BP check required
Last consultation:
   One month ago: exacerbation of asthma
   requiring oral steroids and antibiotics.
   Resolved.

Patient view

Mrs JI is a housewife – she and her family have been patients at the practice since they came from the Middle East to the UK twenty-five years ago. She is active in her local community and leads a busy life with three children, all now older teenagers, and her husband who is a local businessman.

She feels her health has let her down and that she is slowly 'falling to pieces'. She was diagnosed with diabetes three years ago and high blood pressure ten years ago. Her asthma is a problem, and she wants to stop her HRT. She often comes to the doctor for an acute problem – the last time it was for her worsening asthma – or for a single issue like her diabetes, or her blood pressure. So she has made an appointment to deal with a few different things that need addressing. She feels the doctors here never have time really to listen to her, they are always in such a rush.

This time she has a list:

1. Stop HRT
2. More asthma inhalers
3. Check ears, as hearing is bad
4. Check mole on arm
5. Ask about Amin's depression
6. Check blood pressure

118

'Mrs JI – so sorry to keep you wai—'

'I've been waiting for ages and I am meant to be meeting a friend of mine. I have *never* been kept waiting this long before.'

'Yes, I am sorry. It's been a busy morning,' I mumble, following her into my room like a schoolchild in the wake of a disappointed headmaster.

Mrs JI glides along with her nose in the air, like a queen on wheels. She oozes entitlement. The first few times I met her I found her abrasive and arrogant, but I have grown strangely tolerant, even fond of her over the years. That has nothing to do with the presents she brings me at Christmas – usually an expensive bottle of wine in a smart gift bag (though I am very grateful for it). I suppose it's about seeing her vulnerable side, when she was down and desperate with her depression, and it's hard to un-see that. Medicine is a great leveller, a pomposity-pricker. You get to see the chinks in the most important people, and the resilience and humanity in the most humble. I don't take her complaint to heart.

'How can I help today, Mrs JI?'

'It's really not good enough. The waiting room is full of people sneezing, and children coughing and spluttering over me. Why *are* you so late?'

I'm semi-amused that she is talking to me like my mum would have done when I was about twelve.

'Well, I can't go into details of course, but as I say, it has been unusually busy this morning,' I exaggerate. 'I really am sorry to keep you waiting, but I promise I will give you all the time you need.' A dangerous gambit, but it can defuse these situations.

'Anyway, what can I do for you?' All her moaning is just making me even later.

'Well, I have a few things I need to sort out, which we never have time to do. So I shall be upset if we don't have time today. I have brought a list,' she announces in a jokey telling-off way.

(*one minute*)

119

My record for the longest list from a patient is nine items long. I still have it as a memento. But I know colleagues who've broken through the ten-item barrier. I understand why patients write lists – I write lists too. But my lists are usually to be executed over an entire working day, or perhaps a one-hour shopping trip. How on earth people think I can tackle nine different health problems meaningfully in a ten-minute appointment is beyond me. It seems unusual these days for a patient to bring just one problem at a time. A study a few years ago in the West of England looked at more than 200 video consultations and found that on average two and a half problems were discussed in each consultation, with three problems covered in 40 per cent of consultations. More than 70 per cent of consultations involved problems that included several different disease areas. As a result, some practices have resorted to desperate signs in the waiting room saying 'The doctor can only deal with one problem in each consultation'. That's risky, I think, because sometimes people's lists are not lists of tasks for me to do, they are lists of symptoms. Lists of symptoms can be extremely useful for me. Often patients want to talk about several symptoms that they think are unrelated, but which, to a doctor's ear, instantly signal a pattern of disease. For example, feeling thirsty, losing weight and passing urine a lot is diabetes unless proven otherwise. If we restrict patients to one problem only, there's a danger that they might not mention all the clues. Still, many lists are clearly pushing their luck.

The golden rule when a patient has a list is to get your hands on it as soon as you can. Then we can have a useful discussion to prioritise what will be possible in the ten minutes. Patients don't always want to surrender their lists to the doctor though. They hold them close to their chest like a demon hand in poker. We practise the 'patient with multiple problems' scenario in video consultations with actor patients, because GP trainees find it challenging to deal with and it's so common these days. We discuss balancing the patient's and doctor's points of view, and we try out techniques from list-snatching and prioritising with the patient, to thanking the patient for their helpful planning, or even confronting them with a strict cut-off time limit. I devised a scenario with our (brilliant) actors recently to reflect a common variation on the multiple problem theme. Even after outlining the constraints of a ten-minute consultation, some patients get angry because they say they hardly ever come, and they can never get a suitable appointment because they work in the daytime, so they have saved up several problems for me to tackle in this one ten-minute meeting. I can see how this seems logical and saves them time and trouble, but it just doesn't work when appointments are still only ten minutes long. It's simply not fair on other patients who have to wait. With more complex problems, people living longer, and much more prevention work to do, there's a very strong case for longer appointments and more doctors in primary care. But right now we have to make do with what we have – most GPs are already stretched to the limit, working full twelve-hour days. Unfortunately, because I have kept Mrs JI waiting and she is already at bursting point, I don't feel it would be constructive to confront her head on about her fantastical list, particularly given that I am running so late. But I will try asking for sight of her list – that way I can at least acknowledge each individual item, and perhaps even try a little prioritising.

'Thanks for bringing a list, Mrs JI. That's very helpful – would you mind if I had a look at what you've got on it?'

She hands it over silently. She's very slow to let go of it, so we end up in a sort of low-grade tug of war which, in the end, I win.

'OK, let's see. 1. Stop HRT. 2. Asthma inhalers. 3. Check ears. 4. Check mole. 5. Ask about Amin's depression. 6. Check blood pressure.'

'Well, I can certainly get you some more asthma inhalers and check your blood pressure. But you know we have a system for getting repeat prescriptions for your regular medications like your inhaler – just fill out the request a couple of days before you need it and we will have it ready for you to collect here, or at the pharmacy?'

It can be irritating when people ignore the system that most patients stick to. We end up wasting consultation time on the administrative side of prescribing regular medications, which our non-clinical staff can do extremely efficiently.

'Yes of course I know all that. But I've run out of my inhalers so I need more today.'

Ah yes, she has me over a barrel. I can't refuse to give her more 'life-saving' asthma medication right now – even though she probably only needs it right now because she either (a) has been badly organised or (b) couldn't be bothered to order more through the usual channels. I am already typing the prescription as we are talking. Against my own training advice, I have decided to just plough through these problems as quickly and safely as possible. I know her quite well, most of the list items seem fairly straightforward (though not as straightforward as she may think), and by the time I have argued the toss with her, I probably could have dealt with most of them.

'How often are you using the inhalers then?'

Despite my internal annoyance, I am concerned her asthma is poorly controlled with these inhalers so she is having to use them more and more often, which is why she has run out so soon. Asthma is serious and I know she has been admitted to hospital before with it. She needed oral steroids only a few weeks ago. Three people die from asthma every day in the UK, and it's usually preventable. In the emergency department and in the surgery I have been shocked by the speed with which asthma can flip from just 'poorly controlled' to a life-threatening acute attack needing intensive care. To her, this may just be about running out of puffers, but for me it's much more than that. I have done some unilateral prioritising.

'What about the blue one, the Ventolin puffer – the "reliever" one?'

'Five or six times a day?' Normally it would be four times a day for her.

'That's quite a lot. And what about the brown steroid inhaler – the "preventer"?'

'Couple of puffs in the morning?' She's not sure that's the right dose, and is checking with me in the tone of her voice. It's not – she should be using two puffs twice a day; double the dose.

'Are you getting short of breath or wheezy, or coughing much?' All these are signs that asthma is not properly under control.

'Yes, coughing. And wheezing. You know, just a bit tight in the chest—'

'OK, just give me a puff into one of these.' I'm talking over her a bit now. I don't like it, but there's a lot to get through, and I have decided I don't have the luxury of listening or being too empathetic. It's easier to do this with her because I know her and she knows that I *can* be compassionate. She has also slightly shot herself in the foot by complaining about me running late. Personally, I wouldn't start my consultation with a doctor by complaining, even if I felt like it (and I have). I'd wait to the end . . .

I get a peak flow meter from the shelf – it's a plastic cylinder with a graded scale on one side, and a tiny cardboard tube in one end to blow into. The patient blows forcefully into it and the scale tells you the fastest flow of air you can breathe out of your lungs – what's called the peak expiratory flow rate (PEFR, measured in litres per minute). Peak flow measurements can be a useful way to diagnose asthma – in asthma they tend to be lower than predicted for your height and age and usually worse in the mornings, but also tend to improve after a few puffs on a reliever inhaler like salbutamol or Ventolin (a trade name). You can monitor how effective someone's treatment is, too, by comparing their expected peak flow with their actual peak flow (there's less firm evidence for this, but it gives a helpful guide). It's such a simple, elegant device and gives me a crucial objective measure of a potentially deadly condition.

Whenever I use it I think of Martin Wright, the remarkable British doctor and engineer who invented it. He came up with the peak flow meter in the 1950s when there was no practical way to measure lung function – a problem for both clinicians and researchers. I only stumbled across him when I read his obituary in the *British Medical Journal* in 2001. Wright qualified as a doctor in 1938 but with his natural technical flair he became a prolific inventor of medical equipment. As well as the peak flow meter (now used by millions worldwide), he invented the syringe driver (widely used for pain relief in terminal care) and the alcohol breathalyser (which must have saved thousands of lives over the years). Apparently he wasn't terribly motivated by money or professional recognition, and assiduously avoided any sort of committee work. My type of man. The Medical Research Council in the UK created a post for him in which he could just focus on inventing useful things. I wonder if his creative brilliance would have been allowed to flourish like that nowadays. I often teach and test medical students on the use of the peak flow meter – how to explain to patients how to use it properly, and how to interpret trends in peak flow readings over time in the diagnosis and management of asthma. I always try to throw in the inspirational story of Martin Wright.

JI's peak flow is 300: it should be 400. According to the guidelines, a severe acute asthma attack drops the peak flow to less than 50 per cent of the predicted reading. Less than 33 per cent of predicted is life-threatening. So her asthma is not as well controlled as it could be – but she's not having an acute asthma attack. I also need to know the oxygen levels in her arteries (her arterial oxygen saturation or 'sats') – nowadays I can use another little gadget; one that measures oxygen levels just by clipping it onto a finger, like a chubby digital clothes peg. I love gadgets, and this is my favourite. It even has its own neat case. Within seconds it tells me she has an oxygen saturation of 98 per cent. I can relax a little – anything above about 92 per cent is probably OK.

I have a quick listen to her chest. I get her to lift up her top, and start listening at her back. You can often hear more at the back (breasts act like fatty mufflers at the front of the chest – they're hard to eavesdrop through), and it somehow seems more appropriate to start at the back with women, rather than plunging straight into her front.

'Just breathe in and out through your mouth please.' That's the best way to hear the breath sounds as air flows through her tiny bronchioles. I'm listening for the unmistakable high-pitched wheeze you sometimes hear in asthma – a sign of the air trying to squeeze through narrowed breathing tubes. It's like the raspy whistling sounds you hear as the bagpipes are warming up to hit a clean note. In clinical exams, we can't really test whether students or trainees can hear these wheezes because it would be unethical to bring wheezing patients into hospital just as 'guinea pigs' for exams. To get round this, colleagues of mine have tested out using a stethoscope with a built-in MP3 player that plays realistic recordings of various typical breath sounds through the earpieces. It's called the Ventriloscope®. If the patient or actor coordinates their breathing with the wheezing noises (it matters whether the wheeze is heard on breathing in or breathing out) then we can check whether the students are really hearing what we want them to hear. Strangely, severe asthma often doesn't make those wheezing sounds (or ronchi, as posh medics sometimes call them). That's because when asthma is really bad, the airways clamp down so far that the air can't move through the airways enough to make any sounds at all. A 'silent chest' is a worrying sign, and an easy pitfall in assessing someone with asthma. No wheeze – but only because there's not enough air going in and out. There is some slight wheeze with Mrs JI, but none of the crackles I'd expect to hear with a chest infection. The air is ebbing and flowing into the chest nicely on both sides. She is talking normally – she is not struggling for breath.

'OK, that sounds all right. I'll give you some more inhalers, but it's important that you take the proper dose of your preventer – the brown one. OK? That's two puffs twice a day instead of just once a day. That should mean you have to use your blue one much less.' I'm typing as I speak.

(*five minutes*)

'Now, what about your ears?'

'Well, I can't hear properly. My husband says he has to shout at me. It's not normal for me, I normally have good hearing, but I—'

'Is it both ears or just one of them?' I interrupt.

'It's the left one which is worse. They are both bad, but the left one is worse, I think.'

'And how long has it been like this?'

'Oh, I don't know. Maybe. Well. A fair time now.'

It often helps me to know roughly how long a problem has been going on. Or, as medics would say, the 'duration of symptoms'. For example, a headache that has lasted on and off for years rings fewer alarm bells than one that has lasted a few days constantly and that is getting worse. Chest pain that lasts for two hours makes me worry about a heart attack more than chest pain that comes only fleetingly for a few seconds. The story I am trained to tell as a doctor, and which I would tell to another doctor about a case, often follows a set pattern, starting with: 'This is Mrs Smith, she has been getting left-sided headaches on and off for three months.' Or 'Mr Jones is a bus driver who has a two-hour history of central crushing chest pain.' Patients, perhaps unsurprisingly, often haven't prepared their answer that way. Some are incredibly vague ('Oh, quite a long time now'). Some are at the other end of the spectrum, accurate to within several decimal places. Perhaps they are worried that an hour or two either way will put me off the diagnostic scent. I have to listen to their thought processes, in which they often map their symptoms to their own memorable and meaningful life events ('Well, it happened before I went out to play golf last Tuesday – or was it Wednesday? Maybe it was after tea actually'). Doctors have a habit of translating that meaningful timeframe into a purely numerical one. Whenever I go to the doctor I always make a point of working out roughly how long I have had the symptoms, whatever they might be. It saves time.

'Roughly how long – days, months?' I know I'm sounding impatient.

'Oh, probably a week or so?'

'OK, and has there been any discharge from either ear?'

'Well not exactly discharge. It depends what you mean. Sometimes there is some wax.'

'No blood?'

'No.'

'And have you had any dizziness or ringing in the ears?'

I'm ripping through the red flags for hearing loss now. One-sided deafness, especially with ringing in the ears (tinnitus), vertigo or neurological signs, makes me worry about a rare benign tumour of the acoustic nerve called an acoustic neuroma. Ménière's disease can cause deafness, vertigo, tinnitus and feeling of pressure deep within the ear. A sudden onset of deafness (almost instant) makes me think about a stroke or severe infection. The other ear-related red flags are mastoiditis (inflammation and infection of the mastoid bone behind the ear, which can be very serious and lead to meningitis), and cholesteatoma (a rare abnormal collection of skin cells inside your ear which can damage the tiny bones and organs essential for hearing). A perforated ear drum can cause hearing loss too – the drum can't do its usual job of transmitting the sound waves from the canal through to the middle and inner ear.

But the really common causes of hearing loss we see in general practice are ear wax, age-related hearing loss (presbyacusis), and glue ear (fluid in the middle ear, sometimes related to infection). Another way of looking at it is to think of things that block the passage of sound waves from the outer ear to the inner ear (like ear wax, or a damaged eardrum, or a swollen canal, or the thick fluid of glue ear), and things that interfere with the delicate sensory nerve systems that transmit sound (things like damage to the tiny hair cells inside the inner ear, or damage to the auditory nerve itself – both these can happen with age or long-term exposure to loud noises, for example). Doctors like these systematic ways of remembering the causes of symptoms – there's a lot of them to remember and any *aide-memoire* helps in exams. And in clinical practice, of course.

JI doesn't have one-sided hearing loss, it didn't come on suddenly, and there is no pain or history of trauma, or a discharge. That pretty much rules out the red-flag causes or an infection. I'm now thinking this is likely to be either ear wax (I really hope so; it's easy to deal with) or age-related hearing loss.

'Right, let me have a look.'

I open up the matt-black spring-loaded hard case to reveal my precision-engineered metallic otoscope. I grip the brushed steel shaft and lift it gently out of its moulded casing. It's reassuringly weighty. A twist of the metal collar turns on the bulb. I fix a fresh earpiece on the end, like a sniper attaching a telescopic sight. When I first started using it, I was clumsy – holding it too firmly, or too softly, pushing it in too far, or not far enough, tugging at the poor patient's ear, only ever seeing the walls of the ear canal and never the whole ear drum at the end of the tunnel. In my hospital ENT post I learned to use it properly, holding it delicately in a pen-grip, torch part down, using the butt of my hand to stop it going in too far. With a gentle pull of the pinna (outer ear) to straighten up the canal, I now visualise the ear drum directly every time. When it's healthy, the drum itself is a slightly translucent circle, quite beautiful, with ghostly but recognisable shapes behind it. With practice I have learned to make out the outline of some of the tiny ossicles – the three miniscule bones of the middle ear, the smallest in the human body, which act as an amplifying system for our hearing. The easiest to see through the drum is the malleus (hammer) bone, and just occasionally it's possible to make out the hint of the joint between the incus (the anvil) and the stapes (stirrup) bones.

I judge whether the drum is bulging out towards me, convex (a sign of pressure behind the drum, usually from excess fluid or an infection), or being sucked in away from me, concave (from negative pressure in the inner ear). I'm also noticing the colour – the normal pale oyster colour, or the subtle blushing pink of a mild viral infection, to the angry raging red bulging drum of a rip-roaring middle ear infection. Is there a hole (perforation), and if so, where is it? Central perforations, in the centre of the drum, are often thought to be 'safe', whereas marginal perforations on the edge are potentially unsafe, sometimes caused by a cholesteatoma, for example. The trouble is that the photos of eardrums I saw as a medical student were often quite stylised. In real life, all these features can be very subtle. There can be odd bits of white deposits (calcification) dirtying the picture, and lumps of wax in the canal spoiling your view.

All I can see in JI's left ear is a wall of dark brown wax. Nothing else. It's completely blocking the canal, so no wonder she's deaf. I can't be sure there's nothing else going on behind the wax, but the first step is to get rid of it so I can see. The right ear has less wax, and I can just make out half a normal-looking drum beyond it. That's satisfying – a clear-cut diagnosis. If there hadn't been any wax, I'd have had to go on to more sophisticated hearing tests, using tuning forks to compare her hearing through her nerves with her hearing through the air, to see which category of hearing loss it was; a nerve loss or a sound conduction loss.

'Well, no wonder you can't hear,' I pronounce dramatically, pulling out of her ear; 'the left one's full of wax. Totally blocked.'

It's satisfying when you find a plug of wax. Lots of patients worry that it means their ears aren't clean. Many use cotton buds to try to scrape it out. But that's a big mistake. The old 'amusing' adage ENT consultants used to tell us was 'never put anything into your ear smaller than your elbow'. In other words, don't put anything in your ear. The canal is extremely sensitive and it's easy to scratch the lining, introducing infection. Thrusting a cotton bud down it just compacts any wax so that it's even harder to remove. Wax is normal – we all make it and it protects the ear canal from infections and helps to lubricate the skin there. For most of us, wax naturally migrates to the outside and falls out bit by bit without us really noticing. For some unlucky people though, the shape of their ear canals means that wax can get stuck more easily. At the moment, the best advice based on the evidence is simply to use olive oil drops to soften the wax, which makes it easier for it to come out of its own accord. After ten days or so of olive oil drops, syringing the ear with carefully controlled jets of water is then more successful. Without using the drops first, ear syringing can be like firing a water pistol at a brick wall.

'You can get some olive oil drops for that – a few drops each ear every day for the next ten days or so. Make an appointment with the nurse after that so she can syringe your ears. I think that will do the trick.'

(*seven minutes*)

Keep moving.

'And you mentioned you had a mole?'

'Yes, it's here.' She pulls the very top of her shirt down to show me. 'I don't know what it is. My daughter said I should show it to you because you can't be too careful, can you?'

'And has it always been there?' I ask, as I scan the lesion for any portentous signs. I was hoping it might be a simple seborrhoeic wart – a harmless skin growth that looks very like a mole but isn't. We can ignore most of those, or if they're troublesome, slice them or freeze them off. But it doesn't have the typical stuck-on waxy appearance of a seborrhoeic wart.

'I've had it for ages, but it's got bigger in the last few months.'

'Has it?' My ears prick up. I'm looking and listening for the cardinal signs of malignant change in an existing mole – the worry is that they can occasionally turn into melanomas. First, the 'ugly duckling' test – I'm looking for any mole that stands out from the crowd. Uneven colouring is a clue – most moles only have one or two colours, but melanomas often have lots of different shades, particularly very dark or black areas. Any bleeding, itching, swelling or crustiness rings alarms. Normal moles should have a regular shape, usually circular or oval with a smooth edge – when they turn cancerous they can develop a ragged edge or irregular border. Finally, any mole that's getting bigger grabs my attention – and most moles should be no bigger than the width of a pencil, that's about 6 mm.

I usher JI over to the window and pull up the blind to let some daylight in. I have a magnifying glass that helps me to gauge the features.

'How much bigger do you think it has become?' I'm interested in this because none of the other warning signs are present from what I can see.

'Oh not much, but definitely higher – it's more bumpy.'

'And is there any bleeding or itching, or anything else about it?'

'No, not really.'

'Have you had any other problem moles or skin problems?' I'd look stupid if she's had a skin cancer somewhere else. It'd probably be on the computer, but it's quicker and often more reliable to hear it from the horse's mouth, so to speak.

'Well, I have had eczema of course and I needed creams for that. And I had a skin tag taken off from my neck a few years ago.'

Not significant . . . Skin tags are small fleshy growths that hang off the skin. They can look a bit like warts, and they tend to grow where skin rubs against skin or clothing. They are very common and harmless; we usually only remove them if they are troubling someone – perhaps if they're very unsightly or they catch on clothing.

What should I do? I weigh up the evidence as I type up my notes on the computer. I judge that the chances of this mole being cancerous are slim. I refer, in my mind, to a seven-point checklist for assessing pigmented (darkened) skin lesions, based on the sorts of features I've explored. Her mole doesn't automatically score enough for a referral to the specialists. But I am not sure how much bigger it is now than before; probably not much, but she says it is bigger nonetheless. There are no other suspicious features. She has spent time in sunny climates early in her life, which increases her risk – on the other hand, she doesn't have the high-risk freckly fair skin with ginger hair. Should I just reassure her that it's probably nothing to worry about? The trouble is I can't be sure there's *nothing* to worry about. She'd leave relieved and sleep well tonight; I'd probably leave anxious and lie awake. If I'm wrong, there's a tiny chance that she could come back in three months' time with a much bigger cancerous melanoma that has spread or become inoperable. *Daily Mail* headline: 'Negligent GP missed my melanoma'.

Thirty years ago, I suspect many GPs would have had the balls to reassure her. In some ways they would probably be doing her a favour too; shouldering some of the uncertainty, sparing her unnecessary further investigations or surgery, and saving the NHS a few pounds to boot. Very occasionally they might have got it wrong, but society had more reverence for the doctor's role then, and was more tolerant of uncertainty and mistakes. My training was all about avoiding referrals wherever possible, soaking up anxiety. The 'gatekeeper' role of the GP, protecting precious hospital resources, was more prominent. These days, no one can tolerate that kind of riskiness. Patients want to be sure. I want to play safe.

'Well, looking at it, I can't see anything very worrying about it. But I think, given that you say it has changed – increased in size over the last few weeks – we should get it looked at more closely. What we can do these days is get a specialist team to take a very detailed digital photo of it and then send it to a dermatologist for an expert opinion. It's much quicker than going to hospital.'

'OK, yes, that sounds good. And where do I have to go?'

I explain the details and make a note in my red book to fill out and email the referral form for the local teledermoscopy service.

I'm romping through her list.

(***ten minutes***)

'Now let me check your blood pressure, and then you can ask me about your HRT.'

We both know the routine with the blood pressure. She inserts her left hand through the material arm cuff, and I wrap it round snugly, making sure the brachial artery on the inside of her elbow is lined up with the arrow on the cuff.

'Right, are you ready? I'm afraid we can't talk while this is on, as it affects the reading.' That's actually true. It's a godsend when you have notes to type up, or some thinking to do. I type up entries for the three problems so far – the mole, the ear, the asthma. They have to be properly coded so that we get paid correctly for all our activities. It's also vital for any large population-based research studies, which might rely on the accuracy of my data coding. Each entry must follow a clear order: history, examination, diagnosis, plan. Or SOAP: **S**ubjective (blocked ear sensation), **O**bjective (wax in both ears), **A**ssessment (impacted ear wax causing blocked ear sensation), **P**lan (olive oil drops followed by ear syringing). Not too much, not too little. Sometimes the computer feels like an irritating third party in the relationship between me and the patient – pushing me to ask things, telling me to do things, asking me to record everything I do. I have to try very hard not to let it barge in on our conversation.

'Great, your blood pressure's fine: 125/75. Carry on with the blood pressure tablets.' I check the latest blood test results – her blood pressure pills can affect kidney function and salt levels in the blood. We did them three months ago and they were all normal. Fine.

(*eleven minutes*)

'So, we've just got time for the HRT problem.' (We haven't really, of course.)

'Well, I need to talk to you about Amin as well. He's in a really bad way.'

'I'm really sorry, Mrs JI, but if it's about Amin, we should really deal with that in a separate appointment. I'm just aware of all the people waiting outside . . . tell me very briefly what it's about.'

I have buckled. I don't want to risk it being a problem that actually needs our help today. When she gave me that summary of all her problems at the start, I should have prioritised things more carefully, set an agenda. I screwed up, and now I pay the price.

'He just seems so down. You know he is taking antidepressants but he has not got any better since seeing you . . . I am so worried about him . . . can't you refer him to a psychiatrist?'

'This is really difficult. I'm sorry to hear that. But I'm afraid I just can't talk about Amin's care with you – I know you're his mum, but he's now sixteen and what goes on between a doctor and Amin is confidential. I just can't breach that trust I'm afraid. I'd recommend that you get him to come and see one of us, or even talk to us on the phone if he's feeling down at the moment. We'd be very happy to see him any time. Now what about the HRT?'

'Yes, I've been on oestradiol for the last five years. But I have heard about some other type of HRT that's new. I can't remember the name, but I'd like to switch to that one, because this one makes me put on weight.'

I try to listen with an open mind when people talk about pills that make them put on weight. I suppose it's feasible; we know that some medications can do that. Certain types of oral contraceptives, anti-depressants, steroids and diabetes medications, for example. But I suspect that a lot of the time the pills are getting a raw deal, and it's nothing to do with them. To be honest I don't know much about HRT and weight gain. Nor do I know of any new HRT medicine on the market. This just isn't my area – increasingly, women's problems including HRT or contraception are handled by my female colleagues. I tend to focus more on the men's health – erectile dysfunction, prostate problems, and so on. This is partly down to the patient's preference, but partly it's a sensible division of labour along the grounds of interest and gender.

It's very hard to keep up to date with every aspect of medicine – I read medical journals, go to GP update courses, and do online training modules. Working in a big medical school and training GPs means a lot of my work is naturally educational. Professional development for GPs is now big business, and we have to prove in our annual appraisal that we are keeping up to date and providing good-quality care for patients. If those appraisals are OK for five years in a row, then we are 'revalidated' as fit to practise and our licence is renewed. We can thank the mass-murdering GP Dr Harold Shipman in large part for this appraisal and revalidation system – it was one of the recommendations of the Shipman inquiry into his serial-killing career. The process certainly has some value as a review of a GP's work performance, and in devising a supportive personal development plan. It undoubtedly requires a lot of evidence of our activities too: for example, certificates of attendance at training courses, learning from mistakes and complaints, reflection on patient feedback, and audits of our practice. But I can tell you, as an appraisee and as an appraiser of other GPs, it is not designed to catch a devious psychopathic killer like Shipman. I bet the silver-tongued Shipman would have sailed through his appraisals with flying colours – great feedback from patients, attendance at local update courses, evidence of clinical competence, and thoughtful reflection on any near misses or complaints. I suspect the urge to murder more than 250 of his patients might not have come up in conversation.

The challenge with keeping up to date is finding out what you really need to learn about. It's so easy to go on a course about something you are interested in, rather than something you really need to work on. It's also easy to be unaware of your clinical weak spots. So there is a great focus these days on pinpointing our learning needs – for example, through complaints or near misses, which are discussed in depth at practice meetings, audits of practice, or through feedback (we now have to collect anonymised 360-degree feedback from both patients and colleagues). Another popular way is to identify what we call PUNs and DENs. These stand for Patient's Unmet Needs (in other words, I haven't been able to help the patient or give them the information they asked for), which often suggest the Doctor's Educational Needs (what I need to learn about). So here, with Mrs JI, is an ideal PUN/DEN. The patient has an unmet need – I can't advise them about this new HRT. And my Doctor's Educational Need is to update myself on HRT, especially to what extent it can cause an increase in weight, and find out about any new medicines and their characteristics. I'll write that up in my online appraisal portfolio after surgery – or more likely, because I am so exhausted already, the week before my appraisal next year.

'To be honest, I haven't heard about a new HRT. Can you tell me the name of it?'

'No. I think it begins with an H. Or maybe an N. I can't remember. Anyway, it's meant to be very good for weight.'

'OK, well, I will find out about that for you. I can ask my colleagues, and if necessary I can write to the specialists. When I have an answer I'll drop you a line, OK?'

'OK. But I really do need to know about that. Actually, can I just ask you about my hair? I am losing hair in clumps over the last few weeks . . .'

Hair loss. Loads of causes, needs a thorough assessment. Could be a thyroid problem or iron deficiency. Maybe a scalp fungal infection. Maybe alopecia areata – an auto-immune condition. None is urgent right now. Can safely postpone.

'I think we need another whole appointment to look into that properly. It really deserves more than just a couple of minutes . . . can you book for another time?'

We spend hours and hours at medical school, and in GP post-graduate training, learning the key skills of building rapport. Eye contact, echoing speech, mirroring body language, listening carefully, using silence, empathising and so on. But sometimes, when patients seem to be settling in for the morning, the skill we need more than anything is breaking rapport. The specific tricks we learn include breaking eye contact (that's easy, just look at the computer), altering our body position away from the patient, speaking faster and louder than the patient (some people really don't have any sense of turn-taking in conversations), sitting up straighter, handing over a prescription or patient information leaflet, picking up the patient's bag or walking stick for them, or the nuclear option: stand up and go and open the door.

I stand up and walk over to the door. My hand's on the handle . . .

'So I think we've covered pretty much everything on your list – just get Amin to give us a call or come in. I must see my next patient now – thank you again so much for waiting . . .'

(*twelve minutes*)

Chapter 8

Ms JB

(running twenty-five minutes late)

Doctor view

Appointment time: 8.40
Name: Ms JB
Age: 33 years old
Occupation: Call centre receptionist
Past medical history:
    Tonsillitis
Medication:
    Oral contraceptive (combined)
Reminders:
    None
Last consultation:
    Three months ago: viral upper respiratory tract infection. Reassured, no medication prescribed.

Patient view
Ms JB works in a busy customer call centre in town, mostly handling complaints. She doesn't like her job; she finds it exhausting, and she is under constant pressure from customers and from her bosses. She sits in front of a computer screen all day speaking with clients through a headset and speaker. She has taken quite a few days off work in the last few months because of her terrible headaches, and her boss is starting to get annoyed by her absences. He has insisted that she see a doctor to 'get herself sorted out'; she feels that her job is at risk if her absences continue.

Her personal life isn't going well either – she has just been 'dumped' by her boyfriend of six months. She lives on her own in a small one-bedroom flat, and is hundreds of miles from her family and friends at home.

She wants to sort out her headaches, but wouldn't mind terribly if she were sacked from her job anyway. With all the other troubles in her life, she just feels at the end of her tether and doesn't know where to turn next.

'Ms JB?'

My gaze finally settles on the solitary young woman sitting in the corner of the waiting room. She fits my computer's summary – thirty-three-year-old female. As students, one of our seniors would get us to play 'guess the patient's age' during clinic to keep us entertained. I wasn't great at it then, but after years of matching people's faces and bodies with the age at the top of my screen, I reckon I'd do pretty well nowadays.

'Hello – sorry to keep you waiting. I'm Dr Easton.' I say that so regularly that I could sound like a recording on a loop if I'm not careful. Or a medically trained parrot. I'm late but I'm making steady progress through my list. My smile reflects my high mid-surgery spirits.

Ms JB is tall and thin, long-faced and slightly toothy. She is hunched over apologetically and makes only fleeting eye contact as we turn to walk back to my room.

'Have a seat over here.' We both sit down.

'So . . . how can I help today?'

She looks away from me, trying to shield her face. The corners of her mouth start to distort and her forehead gathers into a frown. Her eyes glisten, then close a little. She puts her hand up to her mouth, as if this non-verbal expression of emotion was something she had actually blurted out loud by mistake.

'I'm so sorry,' she squeaks between snatched breaths. 'I didn't mean to cry . . .'

'Don't worry,' I say, nudging the box of tissues on my desk towards her. 'Have a tissue.'

I really don't mind people crying. It happens a lot. In fact I think I welcome it – if ever there was a sign that we have made a connection or arrived at the real issue, then tears say we've made it. I remember group sessions with fellow trainees during my own GP training, talking about what to do if a patient cries. Should we touch people to comfort them? Is that too friendly? Could it be misread? Should we offer tissues? Could that be seen as uncaring – an impatient signal to turn off the taps? Should we say anything at all, or is silence best? Some doctors even cry with their patients when a relative has died, or perhaps after a grim diagnosis.

138

Looking back on those sessions, I can see how they were useful – when you are starting out in general practice it's easy to get tied up in knots over the boundaries between your professional role and your instincts as a human being. But from memory we agreed that the best approach is usually to do what feels natural, authentic. With experience I think that was wise. If you would normally touch some-one kindly on the shoulder and it feels appropriate, then go ahead. If you're not that sort of person, then don't fake it. I'm a handing-over-the-tissue-box type of person. Maybe occasionally I've put a reassuring hand on someone's shoulder, but I don't think I've ever cried in front of patients (though I've felt like it, and I wouldn't necessarily criticise those doctors who do). Right now, I am on the same wavelength as JB – I naturally warm to her vulnerability, and she feels a little silly I think (she wouldn't normally cry in front of a stranger).

After a while, and when it seems that she is ready and able to talk comfortably, I ask: 'So what's upsetting you? Tell me all about it.'

'I just think I've reached the end of my tether. It's these headaches. They're so terrible.' She takes another tissue and wipes her nose.

'It's the headaches, is it?'

I'm naturally drawing on some of the training we're given on encouraging people to tell their story. Subconsciously, I'm in 'active listening' mode; head nodding, a concerned expression, fully focused on her and her story. Echoing a patient's words or a specific phrase is another useful approach, showing I've heard what she has said, and encouraging her to expand on that part of the story. So, headaches . . .

'I never used to get them – but they're just getting worse and worse, and to be honest I don't think I can cope with them.' The admission makes her crumple again.

'OK, don't worry. They can be really awful. Go on.'

My diagnostic radar is already flashing early warnings. Some headaches are dangerous, and the danger signs include 'first or worst' headaches, getting progressively more painful. She can't cope, she's crying, they've started recently for the first time, and they're getting worse.

'I've taken so much time off work with them. I think my boss won't let me have much more time off. In fact he's the one who made me come to see you – he said I had to get it sorted out. I've had the odd headache before, you know, just normal ones, but this is completely different. There's nothing I can do to get rid of them.'

When training doctors, we sometimes think of the consultation in terms of stories, or narratives. One of the champions of this approach is a GP and family therapist called John Launer. This narrative view of the consultation hinges on the idea that patients (and their doctors) make sense of health and illness by constructing stories. In our urge to impose some sort of understandable order on the chaos of our lives, humans instinctively turn to narrative structures. These stories are powerful – they don't just describe what's been happening – an objective reality of illness – they can potentially create a new meaningful reality. They can be all sorts of stories: for instance about who we are, where we are going, or our health or illness.

Looked at this way, the consultation becomes more about helping patients create stories that make sense, that fit, that feel satisfying. Obviously we're not just storytellers – we still have our other doctorly stuff to do. But because general practice is often more about suffering than disease, attending to broken personal stories can sometimes be as helpful as diagnosing a malfunctioning body system or prescribing a pill to correct a physical deficiency. I start to see the consultation as a meeting of two dominant stories. One is the patient's story of their illness; a personal illness narrative. The other is the doctor's story; a professional medical account of what's going on which helps me to organise my thinking and communicate with other health professionals. This professional doctor's account has a clear structure that all medics will recognise: it's a story we've all heard – and told – many times before. First comes the presenting complaint (what the main problem is); then the history of the presenting complaint (the details of the main problem); the review of systems (any relevant symptoms from other systems of the body); the past medical history; the medication history; the family history; and the social history (especially smoking, alcohol intake and occupation). The story ends with a differential diagnosis (a list of possible causes), and a management plan which includes any tests or treatments. This approach has proven itself over many years as a reliable structure for capturing what's medically wrong with the patient.

But real medicine is about people with illnesses, not just the illnesses themselves. It's about the person behind the patient. The trouble is that this medical scaffolding system rips the person out of the story altogether. It separates the person from their illness; it dehumanises the patient's account. So the story JB starts telling me about missing work, being lonely, having the worst headaches she's ever had, all told through floods of tears, eventually translates into: 'This thirty-three-year-old single woman presents with a three-month history of headaches . . .' The trick that we doctors have to learn is to gather the ingredients we need for our professional medical account, while still really listening to the richer, personal account that you, the patient, are telling us. It can feel like patting your head and rubbing your tummy sometimes. Some medical students don't buy the importance of the patient's story – for them it can seem like an amateur obstacle in the way of their professional task. It applies to experienced doctors too – being a slave to the medical story can explain why we sometimes seem less than empathetic, or even positively dismissive of your personal story. Our professional story drowns out your personal one. But without the patient's story, the real-life context, it's very easy to make a wrong or irrelevant diagnosis, or to conjure up a management plan that looks great on paper but is no help at all to the patient. So, in the ideal consultation I let you tell the key bits of your own personal story that you want me to hear, weave it into my professional story, and together we work out a mutual story-ending (a plan perhaps) that feels right and makes sense for both of us.

This is an occasion when I am acutely aware of this narrative view of the consultation. I want JB to tell me about the stuff that really matters to her. I will need to ask some of my medical questions of course, but if I dive in too early, I might lose some of this vital context and possibly some of her trust. I am glad she's already told me how it threatens her job, and about her unsympathetic boss.

'Tell me more about them . . .' I say, deliberately keeping my question rather open, so she can decide what's important for me to know.

'I've never had anything like it. I mean, I have to take the day off work, there's no way I could do my job. And nothing touches it. I've tried paracetamol and ibuprofen, that sort of thing, but they don't touch it.'

'And how much paracetamol or ibuprofen are you taking?'

'Oh, three or four doses a day of each during an attack.'

'And how often do you get them? Every week, every month?'

'Oh, probably every week or so now. It started less frequently but now it's about once a week, yes.'

'That is pretty frequent – but you don't take painkillers between attacks?'

'No, not generally.' Overusing painkillers or migraine medications can be a cause of regular headaches in itself – the so-called medication-overuse headache. The definition includes a headache on fifteen days or more each month, and taking simple analgesics on fifteen days or more each month. Other migraine medications and painkillers can cause it too. Sounds like she's taking simple painkillers about eight days each month – so she doesn't quite meet the criteria.

'Remind me what job you are doing, JB.'

'I work in a call centre. Just outside of town on the ring road, you know. It's really busy; a horrible place actually. Really pressurised. I just sit there all day, hearing people moan at me. And my boss is always on my case . . .' She pulls another tissue out of the box for a final wipe-up.

'That sounds like it could really start to take its toll. OK, that's all very helpful, thanks.' Acknowledging what someone's told me can be a useful gesture to encourage disclosure and build trust. And it really has been helpful. I feel I know what the big issues are for her now. I feel it would be worthwhile at this stage to explore her ideas, concerns and expectations (ICE) – her tearful outburst has made me wonder if she might be harbouring some deeper worry about what's causing them.

'Lots of people worry about what might be causing their headaches. Do you have any particular thoughts or worries on that?'

(*four minutes*)

Headaches are one of the commonest reasons for attending a GP – research suggests that they account for 4.4 per cent of consultations. Healthcare professionals find diagnosing and managing headaches difficult and we worry about missing rare, serious causes. Patients, too, tend to worry about the serious causes of headache, even though they are extremely rare. Typically, patients and doctors worry about brain tumours – though only about a third of patients with brain tumours present with a headache. Meningitis is another worry. Patients often think that high blood pressure causes headaches, although (except in extreme cases) the relationship is usually the other way round. So with headaches, it's well worth getting any worry cards on the table early on.

'Could it be stress, Doctor? This job and everything is really stressing me out.'

It would be easy not to pick up on this cue – to just agree that it could be down to stress and move on with my medical questions. Particularly if I'm running late. But I really need to hear how she thinks stress might be playing a part – in the long run it'll be time well spent.

'Yes, stress can certainly cause headaches, or make them worse. Have you been under a lot of stress recently?'

'Yes. As well as my job, which is really stressful, I've just split up with my boyfriend. That's really been hard. All my friends are miles away – and my family – so it's been a difficult time.'

'Yes, that must be very difficult. All those things would certainly be enough to cause tension-type headaches, or to contribute to your headaches at the very least. But I wouldn't want just to put it all down to stress yet – not until we've explored these headaches a bit more. Is that OK?'

'Yes, of course.'

'Tell me, in an ideal world, how would things be different when you left here today?' I want to know what her story-ending might look like.

'Well, I suppose I really want to know what the problem is – what's behind it. And something to help me deal with the pain and get back to working normally.'

'OK, that's great. So, just to check I've got this right. You're getting headaches that aren't like you've ever had before, they're much worse. You get them every week or so now. Nothing much touches them. You want to know what's causing them, and you're worried about missing time off work because of them. You've also been under a lot of stress lately with the job and splitting up with your boyfriend, and you're a long way from home too.'

She nods. Hearing her own story told back to her nearly makes her cry again. I must make sure she isn't depressed.

'I know you seem tearful right now, opening up about all this. But have you been feeling generally down or depressed, do you think?'

'No, I'm not depressed. It's just been a difficult time. I'm really pretty upbeat and positive normally. It's just talking about it, you know?'

'Yes, I know what you mean. OK. So can I ask you some specifics about these headaches now? Just to help me work out what might be behind them?'

'Yes, sure.'

Whenever I hear the word 'headache', about ten conditions leap into my head like a line-up of suspects to be eliminated from enquiries. Solving headaches always takes some careful detective work. Most are repeat minor offenders – like tension headache, medication-overuse headache or migraine. But there are a few I probably won't see more than a few times in my career – the killers like meningitis, sub-arachnoid haemorrhage (a bleed in the brain) or a brain tumour. I've seen carbon monoxide poisoning from a faulty heater as a cause of chronic headaches too. All these may be rare, but I am on constant alert for them.

144

I'm scanning every word and phrase for patterns that match my medical memory bank of typical headache presentations. Some of the patterns come from years of lectures or textbook accounts, but the most powerful are often from real patient encounters. The stories I generally hear are about 'primary' headaches – common, benign, and not caused by any underlying problem (those are the so-called 'secondary' headaches). I'm talking about primary headaches like the classic migraine, for example, with its one-sided, pulsating, 'behind-the-eye' pain – it lasts for hours, sometimes heralded by an aura, a sense of what's to come, with nausea and visual symptoms, and the patient wants to lie down in a darkened room. Lots of people think a migraine is just a severe headache; it can be extremely severe, but it's actually a specific type of headache, not a measure of severity. Some migraines can be quite mild. Then there's the tension-type headache – the commonest of all – typically described as a 'tight band round my head' but often a rather diffuse headache that gets worse as the day goes on. Stress or muscle tension needs to be there, although patients might not recognise it. It often improves when the patient is away from any stressor (for example at weekends, away from work). Then there are the more unusual 'cluster' headaches, with the watering eyes, nasal stuffiness and episodes of excruciating one-sided pain recurring over two to three weeks, then getting better spontaneously. I need to ask questions that can differentiate one type of headache from another.

At the same time, I'm hunting for the headache 'red flags' – signs or symptoms that should ring alarm bells for any doctor, anywhere in the world. For headaches, the red flags include headaches that are worse in the morning, on waking up, or the headache that gets worse with sneezing or coughing or bending over. Persistent or worsening nausea or vomiting or drowsiness are alarm signs too. These are all signs that there may be pressure in the brain from infection or a tumour, for instance – so-called raised intracranial pressure. Or it could be a severe, sudden-onset headache like a 'thunderclap' (classic for a bleed in the brain, a sub-arachnoid haemorrhage), or a severe headache that comes suddenly during activity, classically during sex. There may be neurological symptoms too, such as weakness, seizures (fits) or balance problems.

Brain tumours very rarely show up with a headache on its own. Unusually, I've cared for two patients with brain tumours in recent years. One man developed a change in personality, which his wife reported ('He's just not himself at all . . .'). Over a period of about a month he had become very disengaged, sometimes not answering when he was spoken to, and unusually quiet. She noticed that he also took more risks when he was driving – he was normally a very careful driver – and he slept for much of the day. Eventually he became unsteady on his feet and developed a weakness on his right side, which was mistaken for a stroke until a brain scan revealed a brain tumour. Looking back he did mention the occasional headache, but it was certainly not a dominant symptom.

The other patient's main symptom was a sense of weariness and tiredness; eventually he started falling asleep at work and was sometimes sleeping up to twenty hours a day. He had a variety of other non-specific symptoms, from breathlessness and weight gain to joint stiffness and sight problems, which made clinching the diagnosis very tricky. But eventually, while on a family holiday, he started to complain that the ground was very uneven and he worried that he would trip. He started to slur his speech slightly, at which point a brain scan revealed his tumour. Again, headache was not his main complaint.

Excessive drowsiness, personality change and unsteadiness are typical red-flag neurological symptoms. Different regions of the brain have different functions – the symptoms of a brain tumour often reveal which part of the brain it is in. Changes in personality point to a lesion in the frontal lobes; problems with balance and steadiness could point to the cerebellum or brain stem.

'So how long have you been getting these headaches?'

'The last few months I'd say. Yes, probably since October last year.'

'And you've never had headaches like them before?'

'No, not like this?'

'What are they like exactly?'

I want her to paint a detailed portrait for me – with as much texture, shading and action as she can muster. Her every brush stroke and pallet choice makes her picture much clearer for me.

'Really strong. Sort of throbbing. Boom boom boom.' She squeezes her hand into a tight fist with each 'boom'. 'I don't know how to describe them really . . .'

'No, I understand, it's throbbing, squeezing. And are they on one side, or both sides? Or all over your head normally?' This is a key question.

'Mostly on the left side, behind my eye, I suppose. But sometimes it's all across the front, here.'

A unilateral (one-sided) headache is typical of migraine, but it can be at the back of the head, or the temples, or even across the whole head. A sinus headache could cause similar symptoms – but the other typical features aren't there. I'm turning down a migraine road now . . . her story is a pretty close fit and at the back of my mind is the knowledge that migraine is one of the three most common health conditions worldwide, along with anaemia and hearing loss. Severe migraine attacks are also classified by the World Health Organisation as among the most disabling illnesses, in the same bracket as dementia, quadriplegia and active psychosis, so her distress levels make sense.

'And do you ever get any visual symptoms with it, or before it?'

'I find that light makes it worse – it hurts my eyes.'

'OK, so you're sensitive to light.' That's me translating her story into my professional jargonised one. A bad habit. Being sensitive to light (photophobia), or loud noises (phonophobia), is typical of a migraine. People often need just to go and lie down in a quiet dark-ened room.

'And do you ever get any flashing lights or spots or lines in your vision?'

I'm interested in whether she has any signs of an 'aura' – around a third of patients who suffer from migraines do. A typical migraine aura lasts from five to sixty minutes before the headache starts. Visual symptoms are the commonest sort of aura, with blind spots (called scotomas) which are sometimes outlined by simple geometric designs, zigzag lines that gradually float across your field of vision, or shimmering spots or stars. Some talented people with migraine have drawn stunning images of these striking visual symptoms – a really useful insight for us doctors. Auras sometimes affect people's sense of smell. But people can also get patches of numbness or tingling in the face or in a limb, or even weakness, or speech problems, so sometimes migraine can be very hard to tell apart from a mini-stroke.

'No, I don't get flashing lights or anything like that. I just find the light sort of hurts my eyes.'

That's a relief. She is on a combined oral contraceptive pill – if she had migraine with aura, she really shouldn't be taking the combined pill; both migraine with aura and the combined pill slightly increase the risk of stroke, so although the risk is small, we should avoid mixing the two.

'And do you feel sick during the headache?'

'Yes, I feel really sick. I've never actually been sick though, just feel like I will be.'

'Is it worse at any time during the day?'

'Maybe mornings now I think of it, but it can come on any time.'

'OK, and does it get worse when you sneeze or cough or bend down?'

'No, not particularly.'

'And how long does the whole thing last usually?'

'A day or two? Usually if I go home to bed then the next day I wake up without the headache – although I feel really shattered for the whole of that day too, so I can't go back to work.'

'And have you noticed whether anything in particular triggers these headaches? Something you've eaten, or drunk; maybe your periods?'

There are so many possible triggers of migraines – the ones I have come across most are wine, chocolate (both of which seem rather cruel), strip lighting or flickering lights, tiredness, periods, and the oral contraceptive pill. Another classic I listen out for is the 'weekend migraine', which comes on as people start to relax, or after excess sleep. But lots of people get migraines without any particular trigger.

'I haven't noticed anything in particular; it just seems to be random. That's the problem, I can't predict it at all. It just comes out of the blue and I have to go home.'

Now's a good time to summarise again – partly to check I've got the story right, but also to reframe her story in a way that helps me to articulate the professionalised account I need to tell myself.

'OK, so just checking I've got it right. You've had these headaches for three months or so, they're coming every week or so, they're throbbing and mostly over the left side of your head behind your eye. You feel sick with them and you don't like lights. Ordinary pain-killers aren't helping much, and the headaches can last for more than a day. Is that right?'

'Yes, that's it.'

'I can really see how that would be upsetting for you – particularly if you're having to miss so much work, and with everything else you're going through at the moment.'

(*seven minutes*)

Empathising comes naturally here. It's an important way to build a trusting relationship, which in turn helps the whole consultation process. Studies show that most patients like their doctor to show genuine empathy and, intriguingly, some suggest that empathetic doctors can even improve some hard clinical outcomes for patients such as diabetes control. Empathy is really about being able to put yourself in someone else's shoes, to understand and share their feelings. It's a sort of emotional resonance. It's different from sympathy, where you may feel compassion for someone, feel sorry for them, but not actually feel what they are feeling. It is a distinction which a team of GP teachers and I struggled to clarify when we were delivering consultation-skills training to doctors in China – we probably could have explained it more clearly, but we were also subsequently told that there is no direct translation of the word 'empathy' in Chinese.

There's also a fascinating (and urgent) debate in medical education circles about whether it's possible to teach, or learn, the skills of empathy. We do cover empathy in communication-skills training, and try to develop students' empathy skills. We talk about how empathy has three main components: the cognitive aspect (understanding *that* someone is feeling a certain way), the affective aspect (entering into a patient's experience and feelings) and the behavioural aspect (communicating that understanding, either verbally or non-verbally). We tend to focus on teaching the behavioural aspects – what to say, what to do – probably because it's easiest to teach. But it's probably not the most important aspect, and there are still doctors who seem short on empathy, so clearly we could be doing better.

Perhaps we could do better at selecting future doctors who are naturally empathetic. But even where medical students start with oodles of empathy for patients, some studies have suggested that medical school somehow manages to squeeze it out of them during their five or six years of medical training (thankfully a recent study has suggested that this might not be quite as big a problem as we had thought).

There are exciting moves to incorporate more humanities into medical education – literature, films, art – to broaden students' perspective and to provide a window onto patients' experiences of illness, for example. There's also been a drive to include in clinical exams some sort of assessment of soft skills, such as demonstrating empathy. In education circles, they say 'assessment drives learning', and medics have so much knowledge to absorb that they are often very strategic in focusing their learning on what they will be tested on. The danger is that students can then learn to make empathetic statements, expressions or gestures without actually feeling any genuine empathy. Their 'empathy' can sound hollow and robotic: 'I'm sorry to hear that your husband died yesterday, that must be difficult for you [*doctor pushes a box of tissues at the patient*]. So, have you had any weight loss or change in bowel habit recently?'

To try to get round this, we often now ask actor patients, or real patients, to judge a student's empathy skills in training and assessments – a patient feeling that they are empathetic is probably the most valid measure. So can we teach empathy? I think we can encourage it, highlight how important it is, and show doctors how to behave empathetically. But I don't think anyone really knows for sure – our empathy measures are still very crude, and it's very hard to design research that can credit teaching as the cause of any improvements in empathy.

Personally, I don't have any trouble empathising. In fact I suspect that I may be an over-empathiser. That may suit some patients, but not all. And there is evidence that over-empathisers are more prone to burnout in medicine, which, of course, is no good for the doctor or their patients. There have certainly been moments in my career when my tendency to imagine, in high-definition, what a patient might be going through has affected my own wellbeing: worrying for them, feeling overwhelmed with responsibility, striving for perfection or certainty for patients, when none of these is achievable.

I remember, as a GP trainee, driving through the English countryside in the middle of the night the five miles back to my surgery, negotiating the alarm in the pitch black, and turning on the computer system. All this because I needed to check that I had given a child the correct dose of penicillin. An overdose of penicillin is very unlikely to cause a problem, but in the British National Formulary (the UK doctors' bible when it comes to medications), it listed central nervous system toxicity as a possible side effect with high doses. I imagined a child having convulsions. The very possibility that I might have made that error made me feel dreadful, and I could visualise all the worst-case scenarios, the effect on the wretched child and its family for the rest of its life. In the end, at about 3 a.m., I discovered that I had given the correct dose, and drove home feeling relieved but foolish, aware that I couldn't sustain a career in general practice if I was constantly worrying about patients and driving back to the surgery in the middle of the night. My golden rule nowadays is to ask myself at the end of each surgery whether any of the people I have seen still worry me, or make me feel uneasy. Then I usually either do some private research on the case, or more often, discuss my concerns with a colleague.

I have subsequently learned that in medicine, somehow you have to arrive at a healthy balance between empathising and retaining some clinical objectivity, a safe distance. I reckon there's an empathy spectrum in medicine, and we probably need people all along its length, or ideally people with the ability to shift along it at different times: from the detached concern of a skilled surgeon during an operation to the close compassion of, say, a GP supporting a bereaved widow. I know I thrive on getting to know my patients over time, building close relationships with some; I find that personally and professionally fulfilling. That's one reason why I opted for general practice and not hospital medicine. As we doctors sometimes say: in hospital medicine the patients come and go but the diseases stay the same. In general practice the diseases come and go but the patients stay the same.

'A couple of other things,' I say to JB. I have just remembered two important areas that I haven't explored yet. They pop up in my mind, much as I might suddenly remember I've forgotten to add milk or ginger biscuits to my shopping list.

'Any history in your family of headaches, or migraines in particular?'

'No, I don't think so.'

'OK, and how long have you been on the oral contraceptive pill?' It's well recognised that the pill can trigger migraines.

'Oh, I think I started it about four years ago, that particular one.'

This reassures me that the contraceptive is unlikely to be the culprit. But I must keep that possibility in mind.

I've ruled out the key headache red flags now, so I am much less worried about this being a secondary headache. From her symptom pattern, the finger is pointing squarely at migraine. But migraine is one of those tricky conditions that, although benign, often masquerades as something more sinister. The sensitivity to light, the sickness, and the headache that is often worse in the morning, are all potential red flags. But if this was, say, meningitis, which can also cause all those symptoms, JB wouldn't be completely well in between bouts. Her headaches wouldn't have lasted several months either – meningitis generally crescendos to a crisis over hours, or days at most. Some people with migraine can seem like they're having a mini-stroke, with numbness or even weakness. Some of the flashing light symptoms in the vision can mimic other serious eye conditions like, for example, a detaching retina. JB is also using a lot of paracetamol and non-steroidal anti-inflammatory medication, which in themselves can cause a 'medication overuse' headache. But I have seen many patients with all those conditions, and her symptoms have more of the character of a migraine to me. This is an example of where I make my judgements on the basis of clinical experience and the ability to weigh up risks. There are useful clinical guidelines on headaches, but this is not a process that can be easily described in a simple flow-chart or algorithm to be followed slavishly by a non-clinician.

(*eight minutes*)

'OK, so can I take a look at you then?'

Examination is important, even though all the articles I've read on headaches back up what I've learned also through experience: that the patient's history is the key to diagnosing primary headaches like migraines, tension headaches or cluster headaches. It's important because I can feel much more confident that there's nothing serious if everything seems normal. It's important also because it's reassuring for patients to know that I have checked them thoroughly and found nothing. If, God forbid, I do miss something serious, it looks very bad – potentially negligent actually – not to have examined the patient. And it can be particularly important if a patient has a specific fear – for example that their headache is caused by high blood pressure. That's why it's always helpful to find out what patients are worrying about, even if their worries seem crazy to them (or me).

A basic general practice examination for a headache would usually include checking someone's blood pressure, and doing a focused examination of their neurological system, including looking at the back of their eyes with my ophthalmoscope to see if there is any increased pressure in the brain. I examine JB's head and neck thoroughly for any scalp tenderness, limitation of neck movements, facial tenderness or muscle tension, guided by her symptom story. In older patients, say anyone over fifty with a new headache, I would also check for any tenderness over the temporal arteries – a cardinal sign of a condition called temporal arteritis, which causes inflammation of the arteries in the temples and can lead to headaches and pain in the jaw during talking or chewing. It's a potential emergency because it can threaten the blood supply to the eyes and even cause blindness.

I'm happy to see that JB's blood pressure is in the normal range. Although the link between headaches and blood pressure is unconvincing (except in extreme cases), a raised BP is hard to ignore, particularly if a woman is on the oral contraceptive pill, which we know can raise their blood pressure.

Neurological examination – particularly examining the twelve cranial nerves coming out of the brain – was always my least favourite examination at medical school. There are twelve pairs of cranial nerves and GPs need to be able to test them swiftly and efficiently, and interpret the findings accurately. Learning neuroanatomy for me, particularly the cranial nerves, was like trying to memorise all the wiring connections in a telephone exchange. I was hopeless. It started to get a bit easier when I began teaching it to medical students. Teaching is often the best way to learn.

In general practice we usually do a focused version of the detailed cranial nerve examination – enough to pick up important signs. A neurologist or a concerned GP would then do a fuller version. I wouldn't routinely test the first cranial nerve (the olfactory nerve, responsible for sense of smell) – I'd only do that if there was a suspicion of some neurological problem that could affect a patient's sense of smell – for example, if I suspected a frontal skull fracture, or a neurodegenerative disease such as Alzheimer's or Parkinson's. In fact the olfactory nerve is routinely overlooked in hospital medicine too – the shorthand in the notes for a normal cranial nerve examination is CN II–XII – NAD. This stands for Cranial Nerves 2–12 – Nothing Abnormal Detected. In truth, I suspect that all twelve nerves get overlooked more often than doctors would care to admit. The standard joke is that CN II–XII – NAD should really stand for Cranial Nerves 2–12 – Not Actually Done. Examining cranial nerves is time-consuming, and to do it properly requires several items of testing kit, such as an ophthalmoscope, cotton wool, and visual testing charts. When the history doesn't suggest anything's amiss with the cranial nerves, busy doctors sometimes don't bother.

With practice, like most GPs, I have learned to do a focused cranial nerve exam in about three minutes. I test the second cranial nerve (the second, or optic nerve), for example, by checking JB's clarity of vision using my Snellen wall chart (the one with the giant letters on), or I can get a rough idea by just asking her to read some small print. I then check her visual fields by sitting opposite her and asking her if she can see my waggling finger in all four quadrants of her field of vision. I'm checking to see if there are any blind spots, which could point to a problem anywhere along the visual pathways from the eye (for example, glaucoma) to the brain (for example, a tumour or a stroke). I check her eye movements by asking her to follow my finger with her eyes, keeping her head still. I check for any flickering or dancing eye movements – called nystagmus – for which there is a long list of possible causes from strokes, tumours and multiple sclerosis to a benign type of vertigo or no particular cause at all (idiopathic).

The beauty of the second nerve is that it is like an extension of the brain. By shining my ophthalmoscope on the back of JB's retina, I can effectively see part of her brain; the end of the optic nerve appears as a small circular dent in the retina, called the optic disc. If there's any raised intracranial pressure (high pressure inside the skull; for example from meningitis, or a tumour), this optic disc becomes swollen and engorged, and its edges become blurred and fuzzy. This is called papilloedema. I'd always look for this sign in someone with a new headache. I've seen it only twice in my career, but I can't afford to miss it.

Learning to use an ophthalmoscope is hard – you have to approach the patient's eye at just the right angle, and wait for the back of their eye to come into focus as you move slowly towards them. Students really struggle to see anything at all – and even after years of experience, the view of the retina with one of these glorified torches is more like a slightly out-of-focus searchlight moving across a giant patch of red sky. You see only a portion at a time, so you have to scan around methodically from one region to the next. Opticians and optometrists get a much better view with their specialist equipment. Apart from the optic disc, I'm looking closely at the blood vessels and for any blotches or spots on the retina – they can suggest high blood pressure or diabetes, for example. It can seem a bit creepy as I inch closer and closer to the patient's face, particularly when they're of the opposite sex, often ending up pretty much cheek to cheek. Doctors have occasionally got into trouble about this because they haven't explained to patients what they are planning to do. It's probably wise to give some kind of advance warning!

I quickly check JB's pupil reactions with my pen torch (second and third nerve); then her eye movements by following my finger (third, fourth, sixth), and then move on to the fifth trigeminal nerve by testing sensation on her face (that's where the cotton wool comes in) and the movements of her jaw. Number seven is the facial nerve – this is when I ask her to make strange facial gestures to check that all the muscles supplied by that nerve are working properly.

'Screw up your eyes really tight. Don't let me open them. Can you frown for me? And raise both your eyebrows? Now clench your teeth really tight and don't let me open your mouth. Can you smile for me?' It's hard to do these facial gymnastics without laughing – we have a welcome, light moment of connection when we both smile at her gurning.

Someone with a facial nerve problem, for example Bell's palsy, will have a weakness of the muscles on one side of their face, causing it to droop on that side. A more central problem with the brain – for example a stroke – could also cause facial weakness on one side. One way to tell the difference between a stroke and Bell's palsy is by testing the forehead muscles – frowning and raising the eyebrows. Because of the way the nerves are wired, with a stroke it's still possible to wrinkle your forehead on the affected side – with Bell's palsy, you can't.

Now for the eighth cranial nerve. I test JB's hearing by whispering in her ears, or I could use a tuning fork. I check the glossopharyngeal and vagus nerves (the ninth and tenth) by getting her to say 'aagh' and check that the soft palate rises and the uvula is central. I get her to puff out her cheeks.

I test the eleventh (accessory) nerve by asking her to shrug her shoulders against my resistance, and move her head to the left and then the right against resistance from my hand. For the twelfth nerve (the hypoglossal), I ask her to stick out her tongue. Is it wasted? Does it protrude straight out, or deviate to one side?

All normal. CN II–XII – NAD.

I complete a brief but thorough general neurological examination, testing her coordination, reflexes, power, tone and sensation in all four limbs. I don't expect to find anything wrong, and I don't.

(***eleven minutes***)

'OK, that all seems perfectly normal – very reassuring. And it's what I would expect given your symptoms. Well, you said you wanted to know what's behind it all – to me, this all sounds very much like you have developed migraine. Do you know much about migraine?'

'Really? Migraines? Well, I know that they're very severe and . . . but why would I have got them now?'

That's a question I'm used to hearing a lot, along with 'why me?' There's a lovely piece of anthropological work that GPs often refer to written by the medical anthropologist and GP, Cecil Helman. Helman studied health and illness behaviour, and one of his great interests was exploring what patients want to ask their doctors when they consult. He came to the conclusion from his studies that when a patient comes to see a doctor with a *new* medical problem, s/he has six questions they want to have answered. These six questions seem to be the same, whether the patient is in London, Beijing, Paris, the Congo or Peru. The questions are: *What* has happened? *Why* has it happened? Why has it happened to *me*? Why has it happened *now*? What will happen if nothing is done about it? What should I do?

We know that patients are often very anxious when they come to see us and they may be too distracted to ask these questions. Helman challenges us as doctors to remember these universal questions and at some point in our consultation to address them, even if the patient hasn't asked them. It is pretty likely that JB has some or all of these questions floating around in her mind right now. She's managed to ask the first one, which has prompted me to think of the others that might be on her mind.

'Well, sometimes migraines do kick in in your thirties – though more commonly earlier in life. To be honest, we don't really know what triggers them.'

As a twenty-first-century GP I often fall down the gap between real medicine and medical research. Patients are increasingly well informed about medical research news, so-called 'breakthroughs', and can brief themselves on most things via the internet. Some bring complicated or challenging medical queries to my door. What causes this particular unusual symptom in me as an individual? Why is this medicine better than that one? What is the scientific link between trigger factor A and disease B? Although I am based in a research unit and feel fairly up to date on evidence and medical news, there are a lot of questions I simply can't answer – not only because I can't be across every paper or study (researchers have worked out that to keep up with the research literature in primary care, a doctor would have to spend more than 600 hours a month reading – and that was ten years ago; it'd be more now), but because medical science hasn't figured everything out yet. Far from it. We're not really sure how statins work, but we're pretty confident that they do. We don't fully understand the scientific basis for all the different types of head-aches, but they happen. We don't know why some people are allergic to certain things and others aren't, and I can't tell you why you weren't allergic last week, but seem to be now. We're not even completely sure of how general anaesthetics work, but they do, very reliably. Likewise, we don't know why some migraines get better when you deliver magnetic pulses through the skin of your scalp – but they do. In fact, there is still a lot of fogginess about what causes migraines in the first place.

I explain to JB the classic features of migraine and how I think they fit in with her symptoms. I am making an explicit attempt to marry our two stories now – her personal experience and my professional account. There's no doubt her current stress levels may be playing into her headaches. I suggest she gets an eye check at the optician and I offer her a leaflet about migraine, and a website address, so she can read all about it later. And then we move on to the ending she told me she was looking for in terms of what to do about her headaches and how to get back to working normally.

When I'm thinking of next steps, I flick through a carousel of options. We teach students to consider all the options first – not to dive straight in with the prescription pad. I'm thinking of things like lifestyle changes, self-help, or the use of time to clarify a diagnosis or resolve a self-limiting problem. And the possible value of involving counselling, self-medication, alternative or complementary therapies, or physical therapies like physiotherapy or chiropractic.

'I think it would help to keep a headache diary for a few weeks, so that you can monitor when they come and gauge if there's any obvious link to a trigger factor. I'll print one out for you. You need to record when you get your headaches and how bad they are, and anything else like what food you've eaten, drinks, any physical exercise, sleep, stress, and so on. It can sometimes really help in pinpointing a culprit. Do you think you would be OK doing that?'

'Yes, sure. And what about tablets? Do I stick with the ones I'm taking? It's just they aren't really working.'

'No, absolutely. I should have said before. You can still take your anti-inflammatories or paracetamol – but I think we should also try you on a different type of medication, specifically for migraines. We'll see if it makes a difference. If I'm right, these tablets should help. They're called Triptans.'

Triptans are kind of magical. Medical science has come up with the goods here. They are not a cure, but they can make a big difference for lots of people with migraine or cluster headaches. Developed in the 1990s, they are 5-HT (5-hydroxytryptamine) agonists, which means that they stimulate the receptors in the brain that the chemical 5-HT, more commonly known as serotonin, stimulates. Serotonin is known to constrict or narrow some of the blood vessels in the lining of the brain, which is thought to play a part in migraines. There's evidence building that it probably also has some effect on

159

nerve endings as well as blood vessels. Taking a triptan at the start of a migraine can really help keep symptoms under control. Triptans don't prevent attacks, however, and shouldn't be taken too early, otherwise they tend not to work so well.

Before I hit the issue button for the usual first-choice triptan, Sumatriptan, a warning comes up on my screen:

CONTRAINDICATIONS – this medication is contraindicated in anyone with a history of:
Heart attack
Stroke
Transient ischaemic attack
Familial hemiplegic migraine

Or currently living with any of these:

Coronary artery disease
Peripheral vascular disease
Uncontrolled high blood pressure

I scan through the contraindications in a second. I know this list, and I am always wary of prescribing triptans, as they constrict blood vessels – always risky in terms of cardiovascular diseases.

'Take one of these when your headache actually starts – not too early, otherwise it might not work. If you need to, you can take another one after a couple of hours, but there's a maximum dose you can take in twenty-four hours.

'There aren't usually any major side effects – occasionally some people can feel drowsy on them, or sometimes feel a bit sick or get dizzy or a dry mouth. If you're happy to give them a go, let's see how you're getting on over the next few weeks. What do you think?'

'Yes, OK, and should I just let you know how I'm getting on?'

'Well, we could meet again in a month or so?' She's not giving me a facial thumbs-up. 'Or do you think sooner?' I am happy to be led by her on this. We can co-create a joint ending to our stories here, one we're both happy with.

'Maybe two weeks would be better?'

'OK, let's make it two weeks – come and see me again then, with your diary, and we'll take it from there. If there are any problems before then, obviously let us know sooner. Now, do you need a certificate for work, for your boss?'

'Yes, that would be really useful actually. Maybe just saying that you think it's migraine and I might need time off.'

'All right, I won't give you a certificate for time off – just a letter explaining the situation and that we're on it. I can always do a sick note if you need one – but as you know, you can sign yourself off for up to seven days.'

'Yes, sure.'

'OK. And look, maybe next time we can think a bit more about the stress you're under at the moment. Perhaps even think about counselling, or something like that? Would that be helpful?'

'Yeah. I guess that would be helpful. It's a bad time right now.'

'So. Are we done? Are you clear and happy with the plan?'

'Yes. Thank you. That's great. I'll see you in two weeks then.'

'OK, see you then,'

'Sorry for crying earlier, I don't know what came over me! I don't normally do that.'

'Don't even think about it. You've been through a lot. See you next time.'

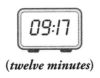

(*twelve minutes*)

Chapter 9

Mr AB

*(**running twenty-eight minutes late**)*

Doctor view

Appointment time: 8.50
Name: Mr AB
Age: 40 years old
Occupation: Businessman
Past medical history:
 Tonsillitis
Medication:
 Nil
Reminders:
 Nil
Last consultation:
 One month ago, viral URTI (upper respiratory tract infection), usual advice.

Patient view
Mr AB has a mole on his back that his wife has been bugging him to see the doctor about. He's not particularly worried about it. He booked this appointment online about two weeks ago, but since then an important business meeting has come up which clashes with his slot. There's no way he can take time off work now. He hasn't had time to ring up and cancel the appointment. He did try once but the phone was engaged. He figures it's too late now anyway.

A light-blue appointment slot on my computer screen. My whole body unclenches and I take a rare slow, deep breath. Seeing a DNA (Did Not Attend) feels like discovering a cheque in the post, or waking from a nightmare. I should be furious about Mr AB DNA'ing. DNAs are a colossal waste when people are scrambling over each other to get an appointment, and potentially risky for other patients who had a genuine need but couldn't get seen. The official estimates suggest that more than twelve million GP appointments are missed each year in the UK, costing in excess of £162 million per year. The traditional health professional line is that patients like AB are to blame for this dangerous wastefulness – either they're forgetful, thoughtless, selfish, or a combination of all three. Much of that may be true. But there is evidence that a fair proportion of missed GP appointments are down to illness (including mental health problems), our own confusing or inconvenient appointment systems, practice mistakes, or patients not being able to cancel their appointment easily. More and more practices are now texting or emailing appointment reminders to patients, and making online bookings and cancellations a smoother process. The debate about charging patients for missed appointments seems to crop up every so often; on the face of it, it's an easy fix, but in reality it would just be too complex and costly a process to administer fairly. The hardest hit are likely to be the poorest and most vulnerable, who are more likely to have to grapple with public transport and less likely to be able to take time off work for doctors' appointments. I can just imagine the heated discussions, the formal warning letters, the mitigation meetings, and the chasing of fines. I do like the idea though of making patients aware of how much their care has cost – their medicines, their consultation, their tests, their missed appointment.

Patients want better access to their GP, so they can see them on the day they are actually ill, and fit their appointment around their busy lives. If I was seriously unwell, with a genuine health emergency, I'd count on the NHS to sort me out any day of the week. But for the more routine stuff, around 15 per cent of patients have to wait longer than a week to see a GP at the moment. Patients often have to phone back the next day, first thing in the morning, to compete in a lengthy telephone lottery for the few available slots. That's far from ideal. Moreover, emergency departments are keen on improving access to GPs in the hope that it might cut the rising number of patients attending their departments with non-emergency problems. Recently, the British prime minister, David Cameron, has made seven-day access to GPs, including evening appointments, a political priority. We could certainly do more to make it easier for patients to see a GP when they want to, but I'm not sure it should be the top priority for a cash-strapped health service, already struggling to cover normal hours.

One of my concerns is that by prioritising seven-day access, without considerable extra funding, patients may lose an even more valuable aspect of GP care: continuity. Continuity is about the priceless ongoing relationship between a patient and their doctor. We have already lost much of the continuity patients and doctors enjoyed two or three decades ago, and it would be a tragedy if we were to ditch what little we have left in the pursuit of ever easier access. Continuity is about the trust you have for the doctor who delivered your children, saw you through childhood illnesses, diagnosed your diabetes or looked after your parents when they were dying. It's about not having to explain your symptoms for the umpteenth time to the umpteenth doctor. It's about having a doctor who understands what makes you tick, your attitudes to your health, and knows about your family and your real life outside the surgery. It's always been one of the jewels in the crown of primary care.

Research shows that continuity of care reduces healthcare costs, provides better health outcomes, leads to more satisfied patients and reduces the risk of hospital admission. The trouble is that when resources are stretched, you risk losing continuity in the pursuit of easier access. With too few GPs and a limit on the hours they can each work, the way to make it easier for patients to see a doctor when they want to is by having lots of different doctors available around the clock on a shift system. So if getting to see *a* doctor when it suits you becomes the most important thing, then getting to see *your* doctor could become much harder. You could see a doctor when you want, but you probably won't know him or her, you'll probably be asked lots of questions you've been asked before, and you risk having tests you don't really need. And although the doctor may have your medical story on the computer in front of them, they won't know the story that really matters – all your ups and downs, the medicines you've tried, the pain you've suffered, the people you care for or who care for you. It's interesting, too, that in pilot schemes trying out seven-day access to GPs, several have discovered that people don't actually want to see the doctor for a routine appointment on a Sunday or in the evening. Some GPs were sitting there, twiddling their thumbs.

To preserve this precious continuity, at the same time as improving access to your GP, we will need more GPs per head of population. There is no easy way round that. At the moment, there is a GP workforce crisis in the UK. At one end of the career path, not enough juniors want to become GPs (many GP training posts are left unfilled) or are opting to work overseas, and at the other end more GPs are choosing to work part-time to avoid burnout, or are retiring early. Other health professionals, like nurse practitioners or physicians' assistants, will be able to take on things like minor illnesses, chronic disease checks and routine home visits, but in the end you'll always need GPs to deal with the more complex stuff.

Some have suggested making better use of technology to offer improved access to the doctor, and I think there is some mileage in that. We could certainly do more email or Skype consultations. Many practices already use email for repeat prescriptions and making appointments, but using it for direct consultations is still unusual. At the moment, practices use email mostly to enable patients to update their doctor on their health, ask for information about medication, or enquire about a health concern. But many GPs are worried by the idea of using email for actual consultations. First, they are afraid that their workload will skyrocket – the ease of email will open the floodgates to the petty problems of those who are perfectly healthy, but anxious. I've experienced that first-hand, working a few shifts as a private company doctor some years ago. People would email me with a running commentary of a developing insect bite, or how their cold was developing. Just because they could. GPs are worried about safety too – for example, missing an important email or the risks of breaching patient confidentiality. And they're worried about losing the face-to-face interaction at the heart of general practice – with email you lose a huge percentage of the verbal and non-verbal communication we normally rely on, not to mention the often pivotal physical examination. I share those reservations. I think we could use technology more, but I don't think email – or even Skype – consultations will ever be a realistic replacement for most of our face-to-face appointments. That's certainly so, based on our experience, with telephone consultations. They're a useful way to give simple advice, and to sift those who need an appointment from those who don't, but so many phone consultations still end up with 'I think it would be better if you came in and we had a proper look at you . . .'

Right now though, a DNA is a welcome friend. It's catch-up time, a little oasis of calm. I check my own pulse – 80 beats per minute: fine. I glance at the photo of my family on the shelf to my right. For a second or two I'm smiling, thinking of holidays or silly jokes with the children.

I take the chance to scan my results and documents. All results from blood tests, X-rays or scans, and those from urine or stool cultures, come back to the practice electronically. We share them out according to how much time we spend in the practice – the full-timers get more, I get fewer. We also try to make sure that we get to see the results that we ordered in the first place – although that's not always possible. I see that I've got twenty-three results to look at, but only five are red (abnormal). The red ones take more time, but red doesn't always mean abnormal. What the computer sees as strictly outside the normal range, I can often interpret as normal: insignificant; marginal; normal for this patient; abnormal but not unexpected; and so on. That comes with experience. So I can't interpret the red results just by looking at the raw numbers. I need to go into the patient's notes to check why they had the test, how it compares with previous tests, what medications they're on, any relevant medical history and so on.

After interpreting them, I need to decide what to do about them – I have a range of prescribed choices from a computer menu:

anything from 'normal' to 'repeat test', 'make appointment with doctor', or 'see the nurse'. Those instructions then zoom through to the reception staff, who let the patient know. Sometimes I need to ring up the patient myself straight away – to start some medication, or even to rush them into hospital. You can't leave a very high potassium level, for example, until tomorrow – there's a risk of serious heart problems. Another urgent worry is a high INR (International Normalised Ratio – a measure of clotting ability in people who take the blood thinner, warfarin): if it's very high, there's a risk of a sudden bleed into the brain. I dread those kind of results coming in to the surgery, and it feels as if they often arrive last thing on a Friday afternoon – I have to track down the patient, then try to pin down the hospital on-call team. The situation calls for urgent action, but the health system isn't always at full tilt at that time on a Friday.

I look at two red results – one a slightly raised cholesterol ('discuss with doctor', and a note made in the records that we need to discuss cholesterol), and one a raised bilirubin ('abnormal but not unexpected' – I notice the patient always has a slightly raised bilirubin level because they have what's called Gilbert's syndrome, a usually harmless condition which can occasionally cause jaundice, caused by a reduced amount of a chemical in the liver, which processes a breakdown product of blood cells, called bilirubin).

Checking results can be a deadly task – in two ways. One, it is monotonous and boring. Long lists of numbers and ranges, most of them normal. Second, it can literally be deadly because, when I'm working through this mesmerising list, it's easy to miss just one abnormal result out of hundreds. A raised PSA (prostate specific antigen, the 'prostate cancer blood test'); an abnormal abdominal scan finding that's hidden within dense text; a solitary, marginally lowered haemoglobin level, flagging up a bowel cancer. One missed number, one missed diagnosis, one devastated life. All of the above are examples I have come across in my career. So I have to be focused and concentrating, thinking of people, not numbers. And like a motorway driver who realises he can't remember the last mile of his journey, if the numbers start to become a haze I have to pull over, take a break. On a quieter morning I would try to chip away at this list of results throughout the course of the morning's surgery – today I'll just have to tackle most of them after I've finished.

I want to take a peek at my documents as well. These are distributed to us in the same way – letters from hospital or from other health professionals such as optometrists, physiotherapists or community nurses; test results; letters from patients; and so on. Often these are a welcome chapter in the story of my patient's illness, perhaps a long-awaited opinion from a specialist. Sometimes they provide a satisfying ending to a story that I started but never finished – what happened to them after I sent them to hospital. I look forward to reading those sorts of letters. But I have to read all of them like a hawk – very often they ask (or tell) me to do something important, but the instructions are buried deep in the third paragraph of a long detailed letter. Things like 'GP to check U&Es after a week' (this is a blood test to make sure the patient's kidneys are working OK after starting a new medication), or 'Please can GP refer patient to nephrologist's to assess kidney failure' (at the moment, hospital specialists are unable to refer directly to another hospital specialist – all referrals have to go via the GP who holds the budget, a surreal game of NHS ping-pong) or 'please prescribe x or y'. The tone of these messages can be rather patronising, as if I am a sort of handmaiden, and increasingly we GPs are feeling that many of the tasks we are asked to do could really be taken on by the hospital team. But, for now, I glance briefly at the eight documents in my inbox, and none of them seem urgent, so I will leave them for later.

I feel good that I don't have too many results or documents to deal with after surgery. And, thank God, I am not the duty doctor today. Poor soul. As well as her normal surgery, results and documents, she has to deal with all the requests for prescriptions, field all the phone calls from patients' relatives or colleagues, and tackle the home visit requests. That's a long, busy day.

(*two minutes*)

168

Chapter 10

Mr GB

(running twenty minutes late)

Doctor view

Appointment time: 9.00
Name: Mr GB
Age: 22 years old
Occupation: Student
Past medical history:
Circumcision
Erythema nodosum (a nodular rash, usually on the shins, with multiple possible causes)
Eczema
Infectious mononucleosis (glandular fever)
Medication:
Flucloaxacillin
Betnovate cream
Aqueous cream
Epaderm moisturiser
Reminders:
Nil
Last consultation:
One week ago, Dr Easton. Diagnosis: infected eczema; Rx (treatment), add Flucloxacillin (skin antibiotic)
Two weeks ago, Dr X. Diagnosis: eczema flare-up, Rx Betnovate (steroid cream)

Patient view
Mr GB is twenty-two and nearing the end of his course as an engineering student. He has been coming to the surgery since he was a baby, particularly for his eczema which can flare up from time to time, although until the last few weeks he hasn't had a bad flare-up for a couple of years. He's been twice to the surgery now and seen two different doctors in two weeks. He knows them both and respects them. He has been given first a powerful steroid cream, and for the last week, an oral antibi-otic to treat an infection of his eczema.

He's back today because the eczema isn't really any better. It's very itchy, and nothing seems to settle it down. He doesn't want to bother them – this is the third time he's been, but he can't carry on like this. His mum has suggested – but he is embar-rassed to say – that he probably needs to see a specialist now.

In a typical morning surgery, I'll see some patients for the first time with a new problem, some regular patients with chronic (long-term) conditions that we need to keep an eye on, and a few who are somewhere along the path of an acute, short-term illness which we are trying to get to grips with. I saw GB only a week ago and suggested that if his rash wasn't improving in a week or so, he should come back and see me.

He's come back. My spirits sag a little when I notice his name on the screen – in one sense, his name spells out my failure. But there's another bit of me that's spurred on by the diagnostic challenge, and by the trust he is showing in coming back to see me again. It's not always disheartening to see diagnostically challenging patients for the second or third time, because very often diagnoses and management strategies become clearer as time passes and with the success or failure of the treatments that I or my colleagues have tried already.

Primary care physicians pride themselves on their pragmatism. We often see our treatments as mini-experiments – when the stakes aren't too high, you can test your diagnostic hunches by seeing if a certain treatment works. For example, if I think a patient probably has asthma, one of the quickest ways to find out is by seeing if the usual asthma inhalers make any difference. This empirical approach to treatment is a common strategy when it comes to skin problems. My rationale goes something like this:

What are the risks of trying cream A if I am wrong? (Low)
What are the potential gains for the patient if I'm right? (High)
And what is the added value of trying to nail a diagnosis with formal tests, which are time-consuming, expensive and often unhelpful? (Not much)

So long as I show my thinking right from the start, and the patient is clear that they are not a guinea pig in a risky experimental stab in the dark, this 'suck it and see' approach can work very well.

I have seen GB over the years since he was a teenager. He had a rough time with glandular fever for a few months, but mostly my colleagues and I have been grappling with his extensive eczema.

There's no cure for eczema, but together we can usually help keep symptoms manageable with moisturisers and steroid creams for flare-ups. At times his eczema was shocking, even to me, with flare-ups that stopped him going on school trips or playing sports. Since he was a toddler, he and his mum have often been in the surgery, at their wits' end over the itchy, scaly redness that had spread across most of his body. It was hard to watch. The word eczema comes from the Greek for 'to effervesce' – his skin would bubble and boil over so severely that he scratched himself until he bled.

As with many patients – roughly two-thirds of sufferers – his eczema had started to improve as he grew from a child into an adult – in fact in the last few years we have only seen him for repeat prescriptions of his moisturising creams and occasional steroid creams that he needed for a flare-up. But two weeks ago, he turned up with what looked like a return to the bad old effervescent days. One of my colleagues – with a special interest in skin problems – had decided it looked like another nasty eruption of eczema and had prescribed the usual treatment: a moderately potent steroid cream to settle things down.

A week later, GB came back and saw me (the original doctor didn't have any appointments free). The steroid cream hadn't helped. The rash was still very itchy, red and had spread further, across his chest, abdomen, groin and limbs. It had an intense redness about it which made me think that the eczema had become infected with skin bacteria – most likely *Staphylococcus aureus*. Typically when eczema becomes infected, it gets itchier and redder – angrier – and the skin exhibits deep fissures or cracks and scratch marks. In one or two places there was also a hint of a gold-coloured crustiness, typical of *Staph aureus* infection. Eczema damages the normal protective layers of the skin, making it much easier for normal skin bacteria like *Staph aureus* to breach the skin's defences and cause an infection. I prescribed an oral antibiotic called flucloxacillin to treat the infection. Flucloxacillin acts against *Staph aureus* infection, and there's usually little benefit in waiting for the results of skin swab samples to check for the bug. If the diagnosis is right, my experience is that the combination of oral antibiotics and steroid cream usually does the trick and symptoms settle down quickly. But GB is back – so clearly things haven't gone quite to plan.

'Hello. Come in. Thanks for coming back – I take it the antibiotics haven't helped much?'

'I'm afraid not. Well, I think perhaps it's like, a bit less red. But the eczema is still there unfortunately, and the itching is like, just as bad as it was.' GB has HRT – High-Rise Terminals, or 'uptalk'; his voice goes up at the end of his sentences, so his statements end up sounding like questions. From his rising inflections, you might guess he was Australian, but actually he's quite posh English. He's a bright, polite young man with a slight frame but a sturdy spirit. I suspect that he is trying to spare my feelings a bit.

'OK, well let's have a proper look at you and see what we can do.' I am feeling a little uneasy, medically speaking, because I am running out of options for helping him now. If it's not an eczema flare-up, and it's not infected eczema, what is it?

I am preparing to reconsider my strategy and ask for a second opinion – either within the practice, or without. I feel that it would be good to lay this on the table right at the start – I suspect that similar thoughts might be going through GB's mind. GPs are comfortable dealing with most of what they see – from mental health and women's health to diabetes and cancers. We're also trained to make sense of the unsorted symptoms that don't yet fit neatly into a specialist box. In fact in our gatekeeper role, managing demand for expensive secondary care, UK GPs only refer about 5 per cent of all the patients they see to other healthcare professionals. We refer for all sorts of reasons: to clarify the diagnosis, to get advice on what to do, or to reassure ourselves or the patient that we haven't overlooked anything. There's always been a sense among GPs – and hospital doctors – that bad GPs refer more, but the evidence says it's not that simple. There's huge variation in referral rates among GPs – even with the modern trend towards national and local referral guidelines – but non-medical factors seem to play an important part. In fact the more expert a GP is in a certain clinical area, the more likely he or she is to refer to specialist care. We also know that doctors' professional attitudes to uncertainty have an effect, as well as patient expectations and pressure from patients to refer them to a specialist.

Most doctors nowadays accept the need for second opinions, and are happy to oblige. While some patients demand specialist referrals as if they were free vouchers for a car wash, in others I sense hesitancy, perhaps a reluctance to question my professional judgement. For them, I find that it can help to broach the subject myself. I don't take requests for second opinions personally, and honesty and transparency are usually the key to success. As generalists, most GPs acknowledge that they can't know about every condition in specialist-level depth. Even if we did, medicine has many grey areas and even the experts don't have all the answers. As medical folk sometimes say: generalists know less and less about more and more, until eventually they know nothing about almost everything; specialists, on the other hand, know more and more about less and less until they know almost everything about nothing. Time and again, research shows that a mix of generalists and specialists is the best approach to healthcare.

'Hmm, let me have another good look and go back to the basics again to check we haven't missed anything. But if I'm coming up against a brick wall, we always have the option of getting another opinion – perhaps from the specialists. What do you think?'

'Yeah, well, that might be, like, a good idea. You know, if it's like, not clear or anything.' I think we have connected here; I sense some relief that the subject has been aired.

'This must be horrible for you. What's the worst thing about it, in terms of how it's affecting you?' This is an ICE moment.

'It's the itching that's the worst. It's just like, all the time, scratching, scratching. And it looks disgusting too.'

Alongside working out a diagnosis, it's important to bear in mind the psychological impact of skin disease. What may be non-serious in strictly medical terms can be devastating for a patient's overall well-being. Acne vulgaris, for example, even when it's quite mild, or the pale patches of vitiligo (another chronic skin condition), can have a huge impact on someone's mental health and their daily functioning. People often try to hide their skin, avoid undressing in public, or develop social phobias. Some patients turn up in surgeries repeatedly with worries about spots that are barely discernible from where I'm standing – but to them, they may as well be a second head.

I could imagine myself as a dermatologist when I was a medical student. I was drawn to the psychological aspects of skin disease. Our dermatology tutors seemed bright and humane, and the visual nature of their craft appealed to my creative side. I think we only had a few weeks of dermatology lectures and clinics in five years at medical school; it was considered a lightweight speciality compared with surgery or internal medicine. But in those few weeks, I think I started to fall in love with skin itself. It would be impossible to create an artificial skin that was even remotely as sophisticated as the genuine article. It's the largest organ in the human body (whatever some members of the medical college rugby club said), a robust and flexible defensive wall separating us from the outside world. At the same time it allows us to interact with our surroundings through billions of sense receptors. It's waterproof but breathable, and has built-in immune molecules patrolling its perimeter. It is an active thermoregulatory control layer, capable of switching rapidly from sweating and cooling to shivering and insulating. It's self-repairing, constantly regenerating, and protects us from ultraviolet radiation. It's a remarkable, beautiful design. If you could make a shirt, or coat, with all those properties you'd be a billionaire.

From a medical point of view, I also liked how it was on the outside. The signs are there for all to see – no prodding or imagining required. As well as the rashes and lesions from contact with the outside world like contact dermatitis or insect bites, the skin tells the inside story – it's a barometer of the whole body's health. Most of the medical conditions we learned about had some sort of skin manifestation – the butterfly rash on the face associated with systemic lupus erythematosus, the typical rash from vasculitis (inflammation of the blood vessels), the ring-shaped lesions in diabetes (granuloma annulare), or the dry skin and thinning hair of thyroid disease. Skin cuts across the whole of medicine.

I think patients often expect me to make a spot diagnosis when they come with a rash. There is certainly an element of pattern recognition in dermatology, particularly for a few classics. The typical pearly lumps of molluscum contagiosum, for example; or pytyriasis rosea, with its pink or red oval patch (the so-called 'herald patch') on the trunk, followed five to fifteen days later by an itchy red rash in the shape of a Christmas tree. Shingles is another – the classic red rash and crop of blisters tracking the course of a nerve supplying the skin but which never crosses the mid-line. Rashes do have the potential for a medical 'Eureka' moment. Once or twice, for example, I have put together a swollen painful ankle joint and a purplish rash on the buttocks and upper thighs of a child to make a diagnosis of Henoch-Schönlein purpura – a rare condition in which blood vessels become inflamed (vasculitis) and which can affect the kidneys and the bowels.

But many rashes and skin lesions do not fit a prescribed pattern exactly; they may be atypical, creams or potions can change their appearance, and they often change or develop over time. They can look different on different shades of skin too. I have seen parents who bring their child in with perhaps one or two solitary spots, to see whether I think they have chickenpox, because it's 'going round'. Well, that's almost impossible to say with any certainty at that early stage of the illness, and with only two spots to go on. It only becomes clear with time, as the rash develops and other symptoms reveal the spots' true identity.

When I was a student – and I teach dermatology students the same now – I was taught that the trick with skin problems is to take a really detailed history followed by a systematic approach to describing what you see.

'So let's go back to the beginning again, GB.' Like a detective on a trail that's gone cold, I need to go back and recheck my assumptions. 'When did this all start?'

'Well, probably about a month ago now. I was at uni when it started, I think.'

'And tell me again what the main symptoms are.'

'Well, the rash obviously, and the itching.'

'And how has the rash developed over the last month then? Do you remember?' It often pays to retrace our steps to the early stages of a rash, particularly when we have been treating it recently, which may have changed how it looks or behaves. Changes in rashes or lesions are often very important – particularly when trying to discern any malignant features in a mole, for example.

'I think it started on my arms, and then my tummy. Recently it's pretty much everywhere.'

'And does anything make it worse, or better?'

'I can't really sleep anymore – it's just so itchy. Even the, like, anti-histamines you gave me aren't helping much.'

'Do you think the itching is worse at night then?' I am taken by his emphasis on the itchiness. I have had to go back to a clean diagnostic slate, and without eczema as an automatic frontrunner any more, I have to think of other causes of intensely itchy rashes. Scabies – an infestation of the skin by the *Sarcoptes scabiei* mite – is intensely itchy, particularly at night as the body warms up, or after a bath. The mites are straw-coloured, oval shaped, and at 0.2–0.4 mm in size, barely visible. They have no eyes, but they have short, stubby legs and long hairs, and the female has blunt spines on her back to help position herself within her skin burrow. The mites burrow into your skin; the itching is caused by the body's immune system reacting to the mites, their saliva, eggs and faeces.

'Yes, I guess it is, yes.'

'Anything on your face or head?'

'No, that's fine.' I'm interested in the distribution of the rash – the bits of the body it affects. Typical eczema affects the flexures of the limbs – the creases of the elbows and knees. Wrists, ankles, neck and face are often affected too – but it can spread pretty much anywhere. Scabies typically spares the head and face in adults, although it can appear there in children. It classically homes in on the wrists, the finger webs, and the armpits. It can affect the bottom and legs, the groin and the lower abdomen. In men, the scrotum and penis can become especially itchy, and in women it can cause itching around the nipples.

(*four minutes*)

176

The fact that skin problems are visible means that everyone can play detective. That has an up and a down side from my perspective. Patients often arrive with theories about what has triggered the rash, things they have been doing recently: for example, patients with poison ivy rash after doing the gardening, or redness and swelling after using a new perfume. Often they've already ruled out a whole range of possible culprits, from biological washing powders to new pets or pollens. Obviously some rashes are caused by a new exposure to something, so this kind of homework is often helpful; we can try to do some sleuthing together. But sometimes it leads to tension between doctor and patient. There is often an assumption that rashes must always be caused by some sort of allergy or irritant – but that is not necessarily the case. Probably the commonest rashes we see in general practice are the non-specific viral rashes that sometimes accompany a low-grade viral illness – these aren't serious and fade over time. They disappear on their own and usually don't need any specific treatment, but it can feel a bit feeble not to be able to give them a neat label and something to make it go away. It's the derma-tological equivalent of 'there's a lot of it about'. Or there's the rash of urticaria (hives), with its raised wheals like an itchy nettle rash, which more often than not is 'idiopathic' (in other words, a condi-tion that arises spontaneously, or for which the cause is unknown). Sometimes there is an obvious trigger like a change in diet or an allergy, but when there is, patients can usually tell me this without any need for tests. Occasionally, it is useful to do special skin or allergy tests. But sometimes a large-scale hunt for a cause just isn't worth it. I do understand that it must be frustrating to leave the case on file, unsolved. It isn't down to laziness, ignorance, or saving money though – it's about trying to act in the patient's best interests, avoiding a fruitless search, and setting realistic expectations.

As well as lobbying for a cause or trigger, patients often want a label for their rash. Although I often want to say (and sometimes do), 'this is a non-specific rash, probably caused by a virus but I can't be sure, and it doesn't ring any alarm bells with me', patients some-times aren't impressed. They want a name. A label. Naming the problem can make it easier to deal with. I learned long ago the importance of labelling – I once witnessed a doctor tell a frustrated patient with a non-specific viral rash that he had 'idiopathic erythema': the patient was delighted to at last have a name for his rash, even though it just means 'redness of unknown cause'.

In a new patient with a skin problem, I usually ask about any past history of skin problems, any family history, and any history of occupational exposure to chemicals or pollutants. But I don't need to go over that in this case – we know GB's history.

'So, to summarise where we are. You've had this rash for about a month, it came on at university, and it started on your arms and spread to your abdomen. It's red and intensely itchy, and it's probably got a bit worse since we've given steroids – certainly no better. And the antibiotics I gave you weren't much help either. It's worse at night-time too . . .'

'Yes.'

As I say this out loud, it jolts me into asking another important question.

'Has anyone you know had any itching or rashes like this?' The scabies mite is usually transmitted from close bodily contact (including sex), or occasionally via shared clothing or towels or bedding. The mites can't jump or fly, so there needs to be fairly lengthy contact for transmission. Scabies often spreads in institutions like schools, universities or nursing homes, where people spend a lot of time in close proximity to each other. And because the symptoms often don't kick in for some weeks after the initial infection, people are frequently unaware that they are infected until they've passed it onto someone else – a neat strategy if you are a scabies mite trying to get around.

'Not that I know of, no.'

That's a shame – an itchy flatmate could have clinched it. But I am now feeling hopeful with my line of enquiry; the picture would still fit very neatly with a scabies infestation. It's notoriously tricky to diagnose and often masquerades as eczema – or even causes it. The typical story is of a patient coming back several times with an intensely itchy rash which has been diagnosed as a variety of other things without success. We were taught that we should always have scabies on our radar (but every specialist and every patient lobby group says that about their pet subject or condition – that's the burden of general practice). Just building up a clear narrative of what happened and when, chapter by chapter, has been extremely helpful. That is why, when patients feel they are wasting their time because their rash has disappeared by the time they see me, I tell them not to worry. We can tell so much from the story and description of the rash, even when it's not there any more. And these days, patients often bring photos of the rash on their phone anyway.

'OK, let's take a closer look. This time can you take everything off except your underpants? Do you mind?'

'No, that's OK; shall I do that here?'

'Yes, it's fine there, or you can go behind the curtain if you prefer, for some privacy?'

'No, that's fine.'

As he starts to undress, I choose to sit down and type some notes into the computer to save time and avoid staring at him.

(*seven minutes*)

'OK, you ready? Thanks.'

Examining a rash is all about very careful observation. I become like a natural historian, or maybe an art critic. In fact some medical schools, including Imperial College where I work, are using art to help students develop their dermatological observation skills. By asking students to draw or model the skin lesions that they see, or to describe a painting in detail under the guidance of specially trained art educators, students can learn to use their senses to sharpen their dermatological clinical skills.

I usher GB over to the window and let the blind up. Natural light is best for scrutinising rashes. I'm just looking to start with – what do the lesions look like? Dermatology has its own group of descriptive terms – jargon really – which, in the right combination, can

179

sometimes bring a particular diagnosis miraculously to mind. Like all doctors, I have been taught to describe rashes and lesions using these terms.

As well as a widespread erythematous (red) rash, I can see and feel papules (raised spots on the surface of the skin), some nodules (lumps deeply set within the skin), vesicles (small blisters) and pustules (pus-filled vesicles). I can also see excoriations (scratch marks scoring the upper layer of the skin or epidermis) and some scaling and lichenification (thickening of the skin, typical in patients with eczema where they have rubbed or scratched the skin).

That's almost a full house of dermatological terms. The main ones missing from this description are macules (flat spots of a different colour from the surrounding skin, like freckles), comedones (black-heads), erosions (partial loss of the top layer of skin), ulcers (total loss of the epithelium) and atrophy (thinning). Oh, and a fissure – a crack or split. And not forgetting plaque – a raised uniform thickening of a portion of the skin with a well-defined edge, like a high plateau in the midst of a desert plain, typical of psoriasis. I loathe jargon, but here is an example where it's actually productive. I can describe any rash using just those few terms, and any doctor anywhere in the world could picture what I was looking at.

Now I want to look at the distribution of the rash. That's just where it is on the body, and any patterns it forms. To be honest, it's pretty much everywhere, but I can discern a concentration of papules and nodules at the wrists and in the armpits (the anterior axillary folds). There are papules in the peri-umbilical area too (round the umbilicus or tummy button), and firm red papules on his buttocks and scrotum when I have a quick peek – with his permission of course. I have a good look at his face, everywhere above the neck in fact. Nothing.

I'm particularly fascinated by his wrists and the webs of his fingers. The scabies mite itself is too small to see with the naked eye, but they say that you can see the burrows they hide in if you look carefully with a magnifying glass. They are like short wavy grey lines. I think I have seen them on one or two occasions, but I am not sure I can convince myself this time. There are definitely papules in his finger webs though, which is unusual in eczema, and classic for scabies. In some areas, particularly on the lower abdomen and arms, there are excoriations – scratch marks – and evidence of secondary infection with vesicles and pustules.

With a decent history, combined with a detailed description of the lesions and the distribution of the rash, I can start to build a picture of the patient's rash and try to match it against the classic pictures of various rashes and conditions. For example, silver scaly plaques on the outside surface of elbows and knees or scalp make me think of psoriasis. Red nodules on the shins make me think of erythema nodosum. An erythematous maculopapular rash (a mix of macules and papules) starting at the head and spreading to the trunk and limbs might make me wonder about measles (although thanks to the MMR vaccine, I have never seen a case except for myself as a child). But a widespread erythematous intensely itchy rash, with nodules and papules affecting the finger webs, axillae and wrists, spells scabies unless proven otherwise. It all hangs together nicely.

This is where the earlier empirical treatments come in handy and make my job easier now – steroids may have dampened down the secondary eczema triggered by the scabies infestation. The antibiotics may have helped a bit to treat any overlying infection. But neither would have helped much with the underlying problem: the mite. That needs a special insecticide treatment.

I ask myself two main questions now. First, should I just treat this as scabies without a definitive diagnostic test? It is possible to check under a microscope for the mite or its eggs or faeces from skin scrapings, and they say that, with skill, you can tease out a mite from its burrow using a needle. But this takes time and dexterity, neither of which I have. The diagnosis, then, is based solely on the history and examination. Second, how is GB going to take the idea of scabies as a diagnosis? Many people baulk at the suggestion that they have an infestation which sounds like a cross between scabs and rabies. It conjures up some sort of filthy medieval plague, and I think people often think it is a slur on their personal hygiene. In fact, it doesn't say anything about your hygiene at all. In 1941, Freidman noted 'the

Acarus scabiei [*Sarcoptes scabiei*] is notorious for its lack of respect for person, age, sex or race. Whether it is in the epidermis of an emperor or a slave, a centenarian or a nursling, it makes itself perfectly at home with undiscriminating impudence and equal obnoxiousness.' It has been irritating humans since at least biblical times and it's also extremely common – there are about 300 million cases of scabies in the world each year.

(**nine minutes**)

'Well, I think I have a good idea about what the problem is. Have you ever heard of a condition called scabies?'

'No. That sounds, like, really unpleasant.'

'I know – it's a horrible-sounding thing. But it's a very common condition that can cause the intense itching you're getting, and the rash as well. You have some very typical features of it – particularly the rash in your finger spaces, and around your lower abdomen there. It often makes eczema worse and in fact it is often mistaken for bad eczema. It can be hard to spot early on. It's also very typically worse at night, which I think you are finding, aren't you?'

'Yes. And what causes it then?'

'Well it's actually a tiny mite – it's very easy to catch from close contact with someone, or even from their clothes or bedclothes or towels. It's extremely common, and absolutely no reflection on hygiene or anything like that – it's just one of those things. It's bad luck. The good news is that it's easily treatable with a cream.'

'A mite? That's gross!'

'I know it sounds a bit gross, but it really is very common. In fact if it makes you feel any better, I had it when I was a student.' Calculated self-disclosure; always a risk but it might help him put it into perspective . . .

'Really? OK.' He nods with a smile. 'And do I need any tests, or should I see a specialist do you think, like you said?'

'Well, I actually don't think we need any tests because, mostly, the diagnosis is based on your symptoms and my examination, which points strongly towards it. There is a small chance that it's not scabies, but I think that's the most likely diagnosis, and the treatment is pretty safe and easy to use. So I would say it's worth a try before seeing a specialist – we can always go down the specialist route if it doesn't work. What do you think? If you feel strongly about seeing someone now, then of course we can do that too.'

'No, it sounds like it's worth a try anyway. So long as this itch gets better.'

'Well, keep taking the antihistamines. I have to warn you that the itch sometimes stays for a week or so after successful treatment. Even up to six weeks occasionally. But usually it will start to improve within a few days.'

'OK.'

'And given all the trouble we've had with this, perhaps it'd be a good idea to see you again in a couple of weeks to see how you're getting on? Obviously come back sooner if there are still problems. How does that sound?'

'OK, yeah.'

(***ten minutes***)

I explain the details of the treatment – an insecticide cream called permethrin is the first-line treatment in the UK, Australia and the United States, according to current evidence. Side effects are usually minimal. I explain that permethrin should be applied twice, with applications one week apart. I talk GB through the details – for adults the cream is applied to the whole body (except the head and neck), including web spaces of fingers and toes, the genitalia, and under the nails. It should be washed off after twelve hours. Close contacts, including sexual contacts, should be treated, and clothes and bed linen should be washed at temperatures higher than 50°C. It's quite a big deal, so I must be pretty sure that it's worth it.

When he leaves, GB seems happy to have a label. The prospect of being free of this itchy rash must be welcome. But have I done a good enough job of convincing him that we've nailed it this time? Is it going to be third time lucky? Will his mum buy into the scabies story? Should I expect a call later, asking for a second opinion from a specialist? I'll have to wait and see.

09:32

(*twelve minutes*)

Chapter 11

Mrs MR

(running twenty-two minutes late)

Doctor view

Appointment time: 9.10
Name: Mrs MR
Age: 85 years old
Occupation: Retired cleaner
Past medical history:
Osteoarthritis
Diabetes Type 2
Hypertension (high blood pressure)
Depression
Chronic obstructive pulmonary disease (COPD)
Cholecystectomy (gall-bladder removal)
Vitamin D deficiency
Medication:
Paracetamol (regularly for pain)
Metformin (for diabetes)
ACE inhibitor (for blood pressure)
Thiazide diuretic (for blood pressure)
Citalopram (for depression)
Ipratropium inhaler (for COPD)
Vitamin D (for deficiency)
Reminders:
BP check due
Diabetes check due
Last consultation:
With nurse, to register with practice. Recently joined the practice, moved from North of England to be closer to her daughter.

Patient view

Mrs MR is eighty-five and has just moved into the practice area to be closer to her daughter. She was beginning to struggle to look after herself properly on her own, and has become increasingly frail in the last year or two. She has lived in the same village in the North of England all her adult life, and was widowed about ten years ago.

She is glad to be nearer her daughter, and understands the rationale for her move, but misses her home and her best friend. She has moved into sheltered accommodation – she has her own little flat on the first floor of a block which has a live-in manager on site and a communal lounge and dining area. There is twenty-four-hour emergency help through an alarm system.

Her daughter has made this appointment with the doctor, partly to introduce her mum to the surgery and discuss all of her medical problems, but also because her mum has had a couple of falls recently and she is worried that she might really injure herself.

The clock is ticking, but it's no good being impatient with Mrs MR, however irked I may feel at her sluggishness. I know this is really an introductory meeting with her and her daughter, so it's important we get off to a friendly start. In the back of my mind, I have memories of my grandfather moving from the Exmoor countryside to be closer to my mother when independent life on an idyllic but isolated farm became too much for him. It's a tough transition for everyone and I know how pivotal a caring and helpful GP can be.

After we've all said hello, shaken hands and swapped smiles, I use her slow shuffling walk to my room as part of my examination. I can check her gait, and sneak in an express neurological assessment. She is roughly oval shaped, like an egg on legs. She is tentative, concentrating hard on each step. Maybe there's a hint of pain in her expression too. She walks – shuffles – unsteadily; an attempt to stay in contact with the ground perhaps, or simply muscle weakness. Shuffling makes me wonder about Parkinson's disease – I'll park that for later. From time to time Mrs MR holds on to the crook of her daughter's arm for security. She's a little out of puff after about five steps, but not gasping for air. My observations map neatly onto the summary I have just scanned on the computer screen. Her rotundity would go well with diabetes and high blood pressure, her painful and unsteady gait might echo her osteoarthritis and Vitamin D deficiency, and the breathlessness points to her COPD (chronic obstructive pulmonary disease).

(*two minutes*)

'Come in then, Mrs MR. Thank you for coming to the surgery. It's really helpful for us – I know it can't be easy for you to get here though.'

'Oh, it's not too bad, dear.' Says Mrs MR with a smile, though her daughter's raised eyebrows are telling me a different story.

'Hello, I'm Jane, Mrs MR's daughter.'

'Well – welcome to the practice! I'm Dr Easton – Graham Easton.' We shake hands. 'How can I help today?'

They look at each other for a moment.

'Shall I say, Mum?' says Jane.

'Yes – you say then.'

'Well, as you know, Mum is new to the area – and this practice. She moved down from the North of England a few months ago and has moved into the Lodge up the road – do you know it, the sheltered accommodation flats? Anyway apart from updating you on all her many medical problems and her medicines, I'm very worried because she has had a couple of really nasty falls recently.'

(*three minutes*)

Falls. I am still listening, but part of my brain is now busy gathering all the stuff I need to think about and do for falls. There are loads of causes, often multiple, some of them serious. There are lengthy guidelines on how I should assess and manage her, and obviously I need to keep sight of this lady and her daughter, and the social spin-offs. This calls for smart thinking and sensitive communication. The Royal College of GPs' motto sums up the challenge pretty neatly: '*Cum scientia caritas*', or 'Science with compassion'.

'The latest one was just yesterday,' continues Jane. 'We don't know why particularly, but of course she could've really hurt herself if she hadn't been so lucky. She used the alarm – so thank goodness she was in the new flat, and not on her own. But obviously something's not right with her and she can't keep on falling like that – can you, Mum?'

'No. It wasn't that bad though. I didn't hurt myself or anything. A couple of bruises maybe.' I admire her stoicism.

'Mum!' Then, speaking to me: 'She'll try to make out it's nothing, but it was very frightening. She's really bashed her leg and her chest on that side, haven't you, Mum?' I admire her concern. They seem to have a close relationship.

'Right. I see. That's very bad luck. So what are your thoughts about these falls then – do you have any ideas as to what's causing them?'

'Well,' says Jane, 'I just think she's getting more and more unsteady. I think she's on an awful lot of pills – aren't you, Mum? – and I don't know whether they're doing her any good really. I don't know, we're just worried that it'll happen again . . .'

Mrs MR chips in: 'Yes. She's worried about me – but really it's only happened once or twice, and now I'm in the flat, there's someone to help . . .'

I now have a flavour of their ideas and concerns, and the gentle, tender tension between mum and daughter on the subject.

'OK, so you fell on your right side. And do you remember what happened when you fell?'

'Not really, dear, no. I couldn't say I tripped or anything. I just sort of found myself on the floor on my bedroom.'

'So what had you been doing just before you fell? Do you remember?'

'I suppose I was getting up to go to the toilet in the morning.'

'And did you hit your head, or lose consciousness?'

'No, I didn't bump my head.'

'And did you black out at all?'

'Well, I don't think so, dear, no.'

'You can remember pretty much everything?'

'Yes, my legs sort of gave way under me and then a moment later I was on the floor. I crawled to the alarm string and pulled it. Thank God it worked, and the warden came to help me.'

First thoughts: this is sounding like a vasovagal attack; a faint or 'passing out' usually caused by decreased blood flow to the brain. The 'vagal' bit is to do with a reflex action of the vagus nerve, a part of the involuntary nervous system that causes the heart to slow down. At the same time, the 'vaso' bit is to do with peripheral blood vessels widening. As a result the heart pumps out less blood, the blood pressure drops, and what blood is circulating tends to go into the legs rather than to the head. The brain is starved of oxygen and hence the fainting episode. There are lots of causes, from emotional stress to sudden drops in blood pressure or abnormal heart rhythms. It's especially common in the young and the over-seventies.

'And just to check – you didn't have any pain in your chest, or funny heart rhythms at the time?'

'No, nothing like that.'

'Good.'

'And is anywhere particularly painful now – worse than before the fall?'

'Not really, dear. My leg's a bit stiff, that's all.'

(*five minutes*)

I'm used to seeing patients who have fallen. Falls in the elderly are a very common problem in general practice. The research says that each year about a third of people aged over sixty-five living in the community will have a fall; half of people aged over eighty. My student training and time in the emergency department makes me focus on the immediate threats to health from a fall. That's why I've quickly gone down the route of checking that she hasn't injured herself seriously – a fractured hip or a head injury, for example. And I wanted to rule out an emergency cause for her fall – say a dangerous heart rhythm, a heart attack, or a seizure.

But there's a much bigger picture I need to address when someone's falling. The evidence is growing – and the message was loud and clear at a recent 'Hot Topics' GP Update course I went on – that one of the most useful things we can do as GPs to preserve the quality of life of our increasingly frail older patients is to prevent them from falling. The human cost of falling is enormous – it can cause distress, pain, serious injury and admission to hospital, loss of independence and, sometimes, death. The psychological and social consequences are sometimes underplayed. Elderly frail people who fall can easily lose confidence and become anxious or even depressed. They can stop socialising and restrict their activities so that they become weaker and frailer and more isolated and lose their precious independence. So, having ruled out any immediate injuries or emergencies (I will examine her properly in a minute) I now need to delve into some of the possible causes of falls in someone like Mrs MR.

'So, it would be really helpful to get to know a little bit more about your general health and your situation in your new flat. It'll help me to get to know you a bit, but also it'll help to work out why you might be falling and what we could do to prevent it in future. Is that OK?' I'm hoping we can address the priority here – her falls – as well as starting to review her medications and her medical history. The two overlap naturally. It's also a chance to build rapport with Mrs MR, and her daughter.

'Yes,' says Mrs MR.

'Sounds good,' says Jane.

'So how are you settling in at the Lodge? What's it like there?'

'Well, yes, it's very nice thank you, dear. Very clean. I don't really know anybody of course – though they all seem friendly enough.'

'Are you spending time in the lounge now, Mum, or just staying in your room?'

'Well, I suppose I'm mostly in my room, but I try to get out to the lounge once a day or so.'

'That's good. And do you ever feel afraid that you're going to fall?' I ask.

'Well, not all the time. But I'm not exactly steady on my feet these days.'

'You said you've fallen a couple of times – is that all, or were there other times?' I ask.

'The only other time really was a few weeks ago, just after I moved in – wasn't it, Jane?'

'Yes, although I reckon you probably fell at least once when you were back in the old house.' She gives me a knowing look.

It can be so helpful to have a relative at the consultation. Particularly with elderly patients, they can help triangulate the facts, fill in the gaps, or add some context. It's great to get to know someone who is the main carer for a patient, too – we will probably have to work together closely. Many relatives who are carers ask for me to phone them directly (with permission from the patient of course) with any medical problems or queries, and that can work well. On the other hand, crowds of relatives with different agendas, or impatient and often absent relatives who swoop in on a flying visit with an agenda to 'sort Mum out' in ten minutes, can be less than helpful. I reckon anxiety and guilt often drive that kind of behaviour.

'You've not had any dizziness, or vertigo?' Worth just checking that she doesn't have vestibular neuronitis – a viral infection that interferes with the balance systems in the inner ear. It can cause dizziness and nausea or vomiting, and usually settles on its own. Also flying through my consciousness is benign paroxysmal positional vertigo (BPPV), a ridiculous label for a condition that can also cause bouts of dizziness, often triggered by movements of the head or changes in position. It's thought to be caused by a sort of crystalline sludge collecting in the delicate fluid-filled balance organs in the inner ear. It's sometimes possible to dislodge the sludge with some specific exercises to manoeuvre the head in relation to the body.

'No, I wouldn't say I've had any dizziness, dear, no.'

'OK, that's good.'

(*seven minutes*)

Now I can hone in on the most likely culprits in an elderly lady like Mrs MR. Falls are rarely down to just one thing – 70 per cent of them have multiple, interacting causes. But I am already thinking that her fall may be partly due to postural hypotension – a big drop in blood pressure when you stand up from sitting or lying down. One of the major causes of postural hypotension is medication. Mrs MR is taking seven different medications – a situation that's so common these days that it has a name – polypharmacy (also a great name for a fictional female chemist). In recent years there has been a huge increase in the number of patients on multiple medications – it's down to a frail elderly population, lower thresholds for diagnosing and treating chronic diseases, and more and more guidelines for the many individual diseases older patients gather (each condition needs its own pills). One in six people over the age of sixty-five are now taking ten or more drugs.

Polypharmacy is generally frowned upon – it can cause a lot of harm with often little evidence of benefit. The more medications someone is on, the more likely there'll be an error in prescribing (one study found that one in twenty of all prescription items are associated with a clinically important error, usually relating to dose and frequency). Side effects and drug interactions are more likely too, and we know that the risk of falling increases significantly when people are taking more than four medications. With each additional medication, the relative risk of falling increases by 14 per cent. When you also consider that most patients would be delighted to jettison one of their drugs (90 per cent according to one survey), it's no surprise that reviewing medicines and even 'de-prescribing' has become a key skill in modern primary care. To be fair, polypharmacy has always been on the radar of those who specialise in looking after older people – I remember how my Care of the Elderly consultant when I was working in hospital more than twenty years ago sometimes used to stop all the medications a patient was on (if it was safe) when they were admitted to a hospital ward. They often felt a lot better for it.

'Let's look at your medications. You're on quite a few, aren't you?'

'Yes, I can't remember them all, dear, I'm afraid.'

'I have a list here, Doctor, if it helps,' suggests Jane. Always good to get a list of what the patient is actually taking – not what the surgery or hospital think she's taking. The two are often rather different. But actually the handwritten list tallies exactly with the information we have had from her old practice.

Scanning down the drug list, I'm spotting quite a few potential troublemakers. We get students and trainees to do this sort of medication review as a training exercise. We call it the paper bag review. An elderly patient, or their relative, comes in with a scruffy old brown paper bag containing all the pills and potions she takes. She empties them out onto the desk. The trainee has to rationalise them, filtering out any unnecessary ones, spotting any potential interactions, getting rid of ones that might do more harm than good. It's a realistic scenario, and really tests their pharmaceutical and therapeutic nous.

Falls can be caused by almost any drug that acts on the brain or on the circulation. Usually the mechanism leading to a fall is one or more of sedation (with slowing of reaction times and impaired balance), hypotension (lowered blood pressure, and vasovagal syncope – a fainting attack), and some problem with heart rhythms (too slow, too fast, too irregular, or briefly absent). People often assume that falls are down to recent changes in medication – in fact they are often caused by medicines that the patient has been taking for a while.

I remind myself what's in MR's bag:

- Paracetamol (regularly for pain)
- Metformin (for diabetes)
- ACE inhibitor (for blood pressure)
- Thiazide diuretic (for blood pressure)
- Citalopram (for depression)
- Ipratropium inhaler (for her chronic lung disease, COPD)
- Vitamin D (for her deficiency)

The prime suspects here are the thiazide diuretic and the ACE inhibitor – both medicines that she is taking to lower her blood pressure. Both – but particularly the thiazide diuretic – have the potential for causing postural hypotension. Thiazide diuretics are water tablets, so they increase the amount of water and salt you pass out from your kidneys. But for high blood pressure it's their effect on widening blood vessels that's most useful. They can, however, interfere with the levels of salts in the blood – particularly lowering potassium and sodium levels, which can cause weakness and falls. There is also a possibility that they could increase blood sugar levels – not ideal in someone with diabetes.

Citalopram – an SSRI (selective serotonin re-uptake inhibitor) for her depression – is also capable of causing falls. No one is quite sure why, because it isn't sedating and doesn't usually cause lowered blood pressure. But the studies say it does increase the risk of falls nevertheless. Her metformin helps to keep her blood sugar levels under control, and whereas some diabetic medications can cause problematic drops in blood sugar, leading to falls, metformin isn't usually to blame for that. Her ACE inhibitor for blood pressure relies almost entirely on her kidneys for safe elimination from the body – if her kidneys aren't working so well, then her ACE inhibitor could start building up to higher levels and have a greater effect on lowering blood pressure, perhaps leading to falls. The metformin, too, can build up if the kidneys aren't working so well, and that could affect blood sugar levels, leading to falls.

So I'll certainly need to check her kidney function, and her blood sugar levels. I check that she's taking her medication as prescribed, and do a quick finger-prick test of her blood sugar – all normal. But proper blood tests are on the cards too. I don't just *think* about Na (sodium) and Potassium (K) salts. I have a *feeling* for them too. To me they feel like dangerous, spiky molecules. We learned how cells need them to function properly – and at just the right levels. But too much or too little can be serious, even deadly. Some of the sickest patients I have looked after have had desperately low sodium levels – or dangerously high potassium levels. When the potassium is haywire, muscle cells don't work as they should. That can affect the heart muscles – if it's severe enough, it can cause life-threatening abnormalities of the heart rhythm. But as I'm keeping half my brain on these molecular murderers inside her, I am also trying to keep the other half focused on her as a whole organism – a real person trying to cope with life. It feels as if, every few seconds, I'm zooming in for the chemical close-up, then zooming out again for the wide 'person' shot.

I'll need to check her blood pressure too – if it drops too much when she stands up, then it may be that her blood pressure medicines are causing the problem. Then we can think about stopping or perhaps swapping one for something else.

I have always enjoyed therapeutics and pharmacology – medications and treatments. It was my strongest subject at medical school. I guess it is where science most obviously plays a direct role in my patients' health. There's something firm to grasp on to, a clear link from drug A to effect B. Unlike people, medications usually behave in a fairly predictable way – there's even a manual (the British National Formulary) that gives me a clear briefing on each one, even suggestions for which one might be best. But they can cause trouble; working out how a patient's medication might be harming them is probably as important these days as working out which medications might be helpful.

(*eight minutes*)

'Looking through your medications, there are a few there that might be contributing to your falls. We'll come back to those later. Now tell me about your arthritis and how you're managing to get around.' We know that arthritis is an important risk factor for falling (along with generalised pain, and other chronic diseases like Parkinson's or diabetes).

'Well, it's my knees and hips. I know I have the wear-and-tear arthritis – what's that?'

'Osteoarthritis?'

'Yes, that's it. Osteo-arthuritis. So my hips are painful when I'm walking and I have to use a stick now when I am out and about.'

'And what about your balance? How's that?'

'Yes, not too bad, dear.'

'Oh Mum, come off it! You're *much* worse balance-wise recently. Very unsure on your feet I would say over the last, well, year or so?' says Jane.

'Mmm. If you say so.' She shakes her head, as a private aside to me. I sneak a quick smile; Jane sighs.

'So balance not so good', I type, staring at the screen, skating over their exchange. I don't like to take sides, but in this case I feel I'm more with Jane.

'And when did you last have an eye test at the optician?' I ask. We know that visual impairment is one of the most powerful predictors for falling.

'I was told to have eye checks regularly – as well as my diabetic eye screening, which is once a year. The last one was a few months ago, I think, and that was fine. I wear glasses of course.'

'Good. Your eyesight's really important. And can I ask a more personal question – about alcohol? We always ask about alcohol when people have falls – even if you don't drink lots, it can play a part. Do you drink alcohol much, Mrs MR?'

'Well, I do like the odd sherry, Doctor!' she says with a coy glance across at Jane. 'I probably have a glass or two in the evening, no more than that. Is that awful, Doctor?' She gives me a naughty, flirty grin.

'Well, why not?' There's a balance to be struck between depriving an elderly lady on her own the pleasure of a glass of sherry in the evening, and giving her *carte blanche* to get blotto every night. This sounds a reasonable amount to me – if it's true.

'Well, everything in moderation, I reckon. If you can stick to just the one, that might be sensible though; what do you think? We know alcohol can affect our balance, particularly as we get older.'

'Oh yes, Doctor. I could certainly just stick to one. If you say so.' I guessed she might respond positively to a hammed-up version of an old-school ticking-off.

'Great. Now, last couple of questions if I may – any problems with your feet or nails?'

'Well, I do have corns on my feet, don't I?' Jane nods. 'But I try to keep my nails cut.'

Something as straightforward as keeping nails short can become a major task for older people, and can lead to all sorts of foot problems and even falls. We have a toenail-cutting service for old people in our area – an unglamorous but essential service.

(*nine minutes*)

I need to move on to my examination now, get some concrete observations, and rule out some of my worries. In particular I want to cross off Parkinson's from my list, and make sure her blood pressure isn't dropping dramatically when she stands up. The two are often linked. I need to examine her chest and listen to her heart to check for any obvious valve problems, and check the rate and rhythm of her pulse. I check her urine to rule out a urine infection – a common cause of falls in the elderly. I'm going to do a focused examination of the balance systems in her brain and nervous system, and then do a general assessment of her mobility and balance called the Timed Up and Go Test (TUGT), which is now recommended in various national and international guidelines on assessing falls. It does what it says on the tin – I have to time how long it takes her to get up from a chair, walk three metres using her usual stick or aid, turn around, and then walk back to the chair and sit down. A sort of geriatric shuttle-run. If it takes her more than twelve seconds, the research suggests she is out of the normal range for sixty- to eighty-five-year-olds, and therefore has an increased risk of falls. If her personal best is more than thirty seconds, there's a more significant risk.

She manages fifteen seconds for the TUGT. We chuckle at the idea of a timed event in the GP surgery, like a mobility Olympics.

'Usain Bolt better watch out,' she says.

I explain what the test means – no surprises, but it does at least confirm our suspicions and put some kind of objective measure on the problem for all of us to see.

Her blood pressure is fine. It does drop when she stands up – as with many older people, the reflexes that help her blood pressure adjust are not as robust as they used to be. But her blood pressure doesn't drop by the prescribed amount within three minutes of standing required for a formal diagnosis of postural hypotension. Like the blood pressure cuff, I am a little deflated at the news. That would have been a neat target for action. It's not a perfect test, though, and I suspect there is an element of postural drop in her blood pressure here.

I quickly assess her cerebellum (the Latin for 'little brain') – the part of the brain towards the back of the skull responsible for coordination and muscle movements. This involves peculiar tests with difficult names, and I have always quite enjoyed doing them because – apart from the terms themselves being fun words – the tests can demonstrate quite dramatic neurological signs. Over the years, I have seen the most florid examples in people who have abused alcohol – the typical signs are an unsteady gait, typically with a wide base; difficulty saying words clearly, or jerky speech (dysarthria); flickering movements of the eyeballs (nystagmus); and a tremor.

I check Mrs MR for all these things, getting her to stick her tongue out and move it from side to side, and taking a good look at her eye movements. I do a rapid check of her cerebellar coordination by asking her to run the heel of one leg up and down the shin of the other. I ask her to walk a short distance, slowly, heel to toe, as a police officer might ask a drink-drive suspect to do. I can check any coordination problems in her arms by seeing if she can move her finger rapidly and accurately between my finger and her own nose. People with cerebellar problems often miss my finger, shooting past it, and move their finger very unsurely.

She giggles through all the nose and finger tests, and clutches my arm, unnecessarily, during the 'police walk'. She's great fun, and I can tell that she's not taking this too seriously. Her daughter smiles at her antics, but I can sense the worry and frustration she feels inside. I try to be light-hearted enough to connect with Mrs MR, yet serious enough to reassure Jane.

'Right, can you just hold your hands out straight in front of you?' Checking for a tremor – particularly the fine resting tremor of Parkinson's, typically a frequency of 4–6 Hz (four to six beats per second). Nothing to see.

'Now, just stand there with your legs together and hands by your sides. That's it. I want you to close your eyes, OK? I've got you if you start to topple.' I rest my arms gently on her shoulders.

This is Romberg's test – a simple way to help pinpoint the cause of any unsteadiness. It's hardly state of the art (it's named after the nineteenth-century German neurologist who devised it), but it can still be a useful test. To maintain proper balance, you need three main neurological systems to be working properly. These are proprioception (your sense of where you are in space, built from special sensory receptors in muscles, tendons and joints), the vestibular system (the balance system in the inner ear and brain), and the visual system. If any two of these three systems are working you should still be able to balance reasonably well. The test is based on the premise that if you close your eyes (losing the vision system), you have to rely solely on the two other systems. So if either of those isn't working properly – say from a sensory (proprioception) disorder or a problem with the vestibular balance systems – you will start to wobble and sway. Romberg himself described the sign: 'If he is ordered to close his eyes while in the erect posture, he at once commences to totter and swing from side to side; the insecurity of his gait also exhibits itself more in the dark.'

Romberg first noted this effect in a condition called tabes dorsalis, a disease caused by syphilis, damaging the spinal cord. I might see it today in neurosyphilis (affecting the bits of the spinal cord that carry proprioceptive messages), but more likely with vitamin B12 deficiencies (which can affect sensory nerve function), or Ménière's disease (affecting the labyrinths of the ear, causing progressive deafness and attacks of tinnitus and vertigo). While the intellectual challenge for medical students is to get to grips with the *causes* of a positive Romberg's test, the practical challenge is to be prepared for the *effects* of a positive test – to catch the patient and avoid a fractured hip or head injury.

My favourite test of coordination has a ludicrous name which instantly appealed to me as a medical student: dysdiadochokinesis. Like most medical jargon, it's from the Greek. All it really means is the inability to perform rapidly repeated movements. I test this by getting Mrs MR to tap the palm of one hand with the back of the other, then turn the hand over to tap the palms together, and then to continue that action repeatedly as fast as she can.

'Well done! That's not easy.' She's managed all the tests pretty well, so I'm not too worried about her cerebellum or her proprioception.

I grasp her hand, and with a manoeuvre combining a handshake, an up-and-down pumping action of her arm, and a rapid twisting to-and-fro of her hand as if wiggling a door knob, I assess the muscle tone and rigidity in her arms and wrists in about five seconds. I've now made a reasonable assessment for Parkinson's disease too – looking for the classic triad of rigidity (stiffness in the limbs, especially a reduced arm swing when walking), slow movements, and a tremor. She has a shuffling gait, which can also be a sign, but none of the others are convincing. Her facial features, which can become mask-like in Parkinson's, seem unaffected.

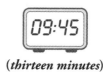

(***thirteen minutes***)

To be thorough I know I should check her feet and eyes properly, but I simply don't have time. I've already been more thorough than I imagine a lot of GPs might have been. That's why I am running so late.

'OK, thanks, Mrs MR. That's all pretty good. I can't find any obvious single cause for the falls – your heart seems fine, and your balance and coordination is essentially intact. One or two of your medicines may be contributing by making your blood pressure drop. But I think there are a few blood tests I'd like to do – just to make sure your sugar levels and salts in the blood are OK, and that you're not anaemic or short on any vitamins. So would you be able to arrange a blood test for those? We can do them here in the surgery – you just have to make an appointment at reception.'

I always feel guilty for asking people to make another appointment to come back another time to have their blood tests. Many patients I see are already annoyed at having had to take time off work for a doctor's appointment (personally, I can't think of anything more worthy of time off work than sorting out your health, and I take time off work to see my doctor or dentist whenever I have to – but that's just me), so to ask them to make another appointment is like a red rag to a bull. When I trained, I took blood tests myself in the consultation, but there just isn't time nowadays. Selfishly, I miss it too – I enjoyed taking blood. Phlebotomy was a skill, a doctorly procedure in which I took great pride. In my heyday I could find a fat baby's vein and steal a sample before he even noticed. Now, I'm so rusty it's usually best to leave all the bleeding to our excellent professional phlebotomists, the clinical vampires of the surgery.

'OK, we'll make an appointment for that. But what can we do about Mum – about her falling? Is there anything we can do to help?'

'Yes, absolutely. This is really key. I think she'd benefit from a thorough assessment at our local falls clinic. It's a fantastic service, they'll do all the tests, and they have a team of professionals there to help with movement, and work on your balance and strength. You'll probably see physios, maybe occupational therapists for any practical adjustments that might be needed in your new flat to make it safer and so on. So it's really worthwhile.'

'That sounds a great idea. Where is that?' says Jane.

'Well, this clinic is based just around the corner, not too far away.' It's interesting that people seem to care much more about where they are going (and particularly what the parking's like there) than who they are going to see. Community-based clinics with all sorts of different health professionals working as a team is the future for primary care. It's always been about teams – not just doctors – but with more and more patients living longer with multiple chronic problems, arranging care in teams based out in the community (outside of expensive hospitals, where patients can get all sorts of problems, like infections or DVTs) is going to become the usual way of doing things.

'I'll send off the referral today and you should hear about an appointment in a week or ten days at most. Let me know if you don't, OK – just as a fail-safe?'

'OK.'

'Lovely,' says Mrs MR. 'Thank you, Doctor.'

'Meanwhile, do you have access to a computer?' I'm looking at Jane, but I glance at Mrs MR – she might be a silver surfer.

'Yes, we have one at home,' says Jane.

'Well, I can recommend a couple of really good sites you can use for excellent tips on cutting the risk of falling – even simple things like making sure the lighting is OK, and that there aren't any trip hazards lying around.' Elderly people are also more prone to fall when they move from a familiar environment to a new, unfamiliar one.

'NHS Choices website has some great information and tips, including some exercises you could do at home for older people. And the charity Age UK has some great resources too. Worth a look anyway.'

'Yes, we will. Thank you, doctor,' says Jane.

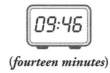

(fourteen minutes)

I've forgotten to alter her medications. I suggest stopping the thiazide – it may help, and it's unlikely to cause any major problems. We'll keep an eye on her blood pressure.

'Is that all OK then? Everything clear? And come and see me again to discuss those results and check how you're doing in a month – will that be OK?'

It's sensible to keep an eye on someone like Mrs MR; in fact the guidelines suggest a review in a month for patients at high risk of falling, and there is huge value in us getting to know each other, building a bond, and showing her daughter too that we're here for the duration. I can finish off some of the things I haven't managed to do this time, too.

'Yes, thank you so much, Doctor. That's great. And we'll see you again in a month or so.'

'Thank you, dear,' says Mrs MR. 'I'll get into training for that walking test – maybe I'll break my record next time!' She winks at me.

'I'm sure you will, Mrs MR. I look forward to seeing that,' I say through a smile.

Jane shakes her head and rolls her eyes at me in fake despair.

Big red book out. 'Refer to falls clinic.'

I reckon that went pretty well. I think I've made a genuine connection with Mrs MR and her daughter and I've done a reasonable assessment of her falls. I've offered them support. I haven't been able to pinpoint a single cause, but I've ruled out some of the important ones, organised tests to exclude some others, and come up with a management plan that they're both happy with. In the end, it should mean she's less likely to fall in the future. It's taken me fifteen minutes, but it was worth it. They don't all go like that.

(*fifteen minutes*)

Chapter 12

Mr EB

(running twenty-eight minutes late)

Doctor view

Appointment time: 9.20
Name: Mr EB
Age: 47 years old
Occupation: Self-employed designer
Past medical history:
    Sinusitis
    Appendicectomy
    Hernia repair
Medication:
    Nil
Reminders:
    None
Last consultation:
    Saw me six weeks ago with acute sinusitis, prescribed amoxicillin 500 mg TDS. Six consultations for a variety of minor illnesses over the last year or so.

Patient view

Mr EB is a 47-year-old designer. He is married with two children, a girl aged fifteen and a boy aged twelve. He feels as though he has hit some kind of mid-life health barrier, and everything is falling apart. He is constantly tired, often needing to take naps during the day, which interferes with his work. He just hasn't had any energy over the last three months or so. He seems to have had several infections recently, more than usual for him. His eyesight has deteriorated over the last couple of years, and he gets a constant stream of muscular or joint problems, from tennis elbow to painful knees. He isn't sleeping brilliantly either, and has had a lot of headaches recently.

He is concerned that something must be underlying all these problems as, up until about a year ago, he felt very healthy. None of the doctors has been able to sort out any of his complaints. He suspects this time the doctor might fob him off with 'stress' as a reason – his wife was given the same label and it turned out to be an underactive thyroid gland.

'Hello, sorry to keep you waiting. I'm Dr Easton . . . I don't think we've met before, have we?'

'Yes, we have actually, a few weeks ago – I came about my sinuses.'

'Oh yes, of course. Sorry.' Really bad start. Not a great way to build rapport – the first task in any consultation. I must remember not to use that line again . . . or at least to always scan the notes before the patient comes in. I'm rushing to keep up, cutting corners. I secretly check my pulse; I estimate about 90 beats per minute. Too fast.

'Of course – I recognise you now, yes.' I am digging. 'So . . . how can I help?' I ask, hoping to move swiftly on.

'Well, where do I start – how long have you got!?' It's a flippant, jokey line, but right now, running nearly half an hour late, it feels like a rather unfunny threat.

'Well, we have ten minutes,' I say, smiling, but hoping the message is clear. I am struggling to feel any natural rapport building here. He's direct, unsmiling, and there's not much eye contact going on.

'Yes, right. Well, for the last, well, few months I suppose, I just haven't been feeling right. I've had so many things, just one after the other, and that's not like me. I just feel so tired all the time. Utterly exhausted. So, I came to see you about my sinuses about six weeks ago, and you gave me some antibiotics, but that hasn't completely gone away. And I just seem to be getting infection after infection. I've been here loads of times with coughs, sore throats, colds – you know, much more than I used to. Actually I do need to ask you about my sore throat – that just doesn't feel right and I've constantly got these lymph nodes in my neck recently which isn't normal – is it? And then the whole tiredness thing – I just feel absolutely knack-ered all the time – and it's not stress because I really am not stressed at the moment – there's nothing remotely stressful going on for me at the moment, in fact I should be feeling better than ever because, you know, my work's going well, family's good, money's fine. One doctor said I was overweight but that's not going to make me feel like this, is it, suddenly, just in a few months? And that's another thing actually – I keep getting muscular problems or joint pains – I came about tennis elbow a few months ago (that's still not right, by the way) – but until about, oh, a year ago, I had never had any problems like that at all. I never used to get those sort of problems. My skin is really dry too – both my elbows, my legs down here – and I'm getting more headaches now than I used to as well . . . like at least one a week, which is much more frequent than I have ever experienced. And with this absolute exhaustion, you know, something's just not right.'

With every sentence he fires another problem at me, like an endless onslaught of enemy soldiers going over the top. As soon I shoot one down, up pops another. I'm a little overwhelmed, and starting to feel like an untrained conscript. Maybe I'm a hopeless doctor, unable to help the patient; I should have read the right articles or been on a better course. When I was training thirty years ago, we might have labelled him a 'heartsink' patient; according to Tom O'Dowd, an academic GP writing in the *British Journal of General Practice* in 1988, these are the patients who 'exasperate, defeat and overwhelm their doctors by their behaviour'. An earlier paper, from 1978, even described some regular heartsinks as 'hateful patients' and described four main stereotypes. There's the Dependent Clinger, who's grateful for their care but keeps coming back with a new array of symptoms; the Entitled Demander, who is full of complaints and sees the doctor as a barrier to getting the services they want; the Manipulative Help-Rejecter, who returns repeatedly to tell the doctor that the treatment isn't working, and any suggestions of 'Why don't you try . . .' are met with 'Yes, but . . .'; and finally the Self-Destructive Denier, who may well suffer from serious disease but makes no changes in their lifestyle and seems hell-bent on rejecting any attempts to help them. More than three decades later this stereotyping might seem shockingly outdated: a politically incorrect judgement about a patient, and a denial of the role of the doctor in difficult encounters. On the other hand, it's an honest description of how some patients can occasionally make you feel as a GP, and the paper was an early attempt to help doctors care for those patients who filled them with dread.

What I find interesting is how GPs' understanding of the heartsink phenomenon has evolved. A 1995 study in the same journal looked at the contribution of the doctor in these troubling encounters. It found that doctors were likely to report more heartsink patients if they felt overworked, if they were unsatisfied with their job, or if they lacked training in communication skills or relevant postgraduate qualifications. Nowadays you'll still hear the term 'heartsink' in surgeries up and down the land, but we talk much more about heartsink consultations, which involve both a patient and a doctor. And as a result, we've developed more constructive approaches to dealing with them. For example, we accept that we can't diagnose or cure all our patients – we see lots of patients with symptoms that can't be explained medically (fatigue is one). Simply lowering our often unrealistic expectations of consultations can soften the heartsink feeling in us (patients are often more aware of our limitations than we are). Meeting regularly in peer support groups, keeping reflective diaries, and sharing care with another doctor can all help, too.

Another approach, which I think I'll try now, is based on an awareness of how a patient is making me feel, and how this often reflects the patient's own feelings. In other words, a patient who makes me feel helpless and overwhelmed may be feeling helpless and overwhelmed themselves. I'm just picking up his overwhelmed 'vibes'. Reflecting that back to the patient can sometimes offer him or her useful new insights. It also softens my conviction that I really am an incompetent doctor. It's important to be aware of my limitations, of course (and I am acutely aware of those, including my often unhelpful urge to 'sort everything out' – a recipe for sustained disappointment), but to believe that you're useless is an unhelpful standpoint by any measure. The trouble is that, as you can imagine, batting this tidal wave of despond and angst back at him while wrapping it up as if it were a precious gift is a delicate skill.

'OK. That's quite a list there, isn't it? The tiredness, the headaches, muscle and joint problems, skin dryness, recurrent infections – I can imagine that's an awful lot to deal with. I'm just wondering if it all gets . . . overwhelming sometimes?'

I'm couching this as a suggestion – there's an upwards intonation at the end of the sentence. My version of HRT (High-Rise Terminals).

It's a gamble; I'm aware we haven't got off to a roaring start, and this could backfire by putting him on the spot. But I decide it's worth a last-ditch roll of the rapport dice. He can reject it, and that's fine. But often patients only partially reject my proposal – perhaps correcting a small aspect of it and accepting the bulk. Or they rebuff it completely at the time, in that particular consultation, but it simmers away enough to help them move on emotionally the next time I see them. It's also a nice way to summarise what he has told me – to show him I've heard, and give him a chance to put me right, if necessary.

'Yes, it is a lot to deal with. It's just all come at once, you know, and it's hard to understand why all this stuff is happening now?'

'I can imagine, and you said that you felt "something just isn't right" earlier.' This is going better now. I picked up on this 'cue' previously but have only just had the chance to offer it back to him. 'It's really hard when there's no clear answer, no single unifying explanation for everything.' I leave it at that: a statement. I want to see how he picks this up.

'Yes, well I guess that's why I have come today, to see if there is an explanation for it all. Maybe there isn't – maybe I'm just getting to that age. But it just seems weird, that's all.'

I feel like we have made some headway. I have dropped in the suggestion that there may be no overarching explanation that ties all his symptoms neatly together, and he hasn't rejected it out of hand. Of course there may be – and that possibility looms large in my mind. But often there isn't. We only make a clear diagnosis in less than half of all patients with fatigue, and many of those diagnoses are really just descriptive ones such as 'stress' or synonyms for fatigue itself. Although studies suggest that patients do understand that there might not be an identifiable cause for their fatigue, patients' and doctors' beliefs are sometimes mismatched, with more doctors than patients considering the problem to be psychological. With the benefit of what medics call the 'retrospectoscope' (and what everyone else calls hindsight), over the years many patients have turned out to have significant causes for their tiredness, from anaemia or depression to chronic fatigue or underactive thyroid glands. My mother is an example. She is a slim, fit regular walker, but during a family holiday in Wales a few years ago we noticed that she was becoming more and more fatigued and out of breath walking up gentle slopes. I persuaded her to go to the GP – the blood tests showed she was anaemic and the cause turned out to be an early bowel cancer. I'm pleased to say that she has made an excellent recovery. That is the essence of the GP's challenge. Fatigue is a normal part of everyday life, but it can occasionally be a sign of disease, and sometimes serious illness.

Between 5 and 7 per cent of all consultations has fatigue as a main complaint, a figure that is remarkably consistent across all Western countries, and over time. The only more common complaint in primary care is a cough. The proportion of patients who present with fatigue as an add-on complaint is almost three times higher. I guess that's why we have a ready-made acronym for it: 'TATT', which stands for 'tired all the time'. It's one of the few acronyms we still write in patients' records (in fact it's an official code in most medical record systems) – most of the others, often offensive (like TUBE: 'totally unnecessary breast examination', NFN: 'normal for Norfolk', or FLK: 'funny-looking kid') died a death decades ago when it became possible for patients to access their own records. But TATT somehow doesn't seem offensive; I could be wrong, but it's not meant in a derogatory sense; it's how patients tend to describe what they're feeling, and it's useful shorthand for a very common problem.

Mr EB has even suggested that it might all be 'one of those things' – perhaps just down to age, or what we call 'Anno Domini'. On reflection, this has been a satisfactory start; managing expectations is often a key step in modern primary care. And I am not feeling quite so much like a reluctant conscript stuck in the mud. My mission doesn't seem so daunting now. I charge forward, bayonet fixed.

'So what would you say is troubling you most?' This is a handy question to help people focus when they bring long lists of problems. I am happy for him to steer the consultation. Zooming through my mind are a few conditions that might explain all or many of his symptoms, and I'll bear those in mind as we talk, but right now a focus would be helpful.

'Well, I suppose it's the tiredness. You know, just constant tiredness. I have to nap for an hour or so some days – luckily, I can because I work from home, but it does mean I am not getting much work done and that's a problem because clients get annoyed and in fact I have lost a couple of projects actually because of that.'

'Right, I see. Sorry to hear that. And when you say tiredness, what do you mean by that? Do you mean weak and short of energy, for example, or more drowsy and not refreshed when you wake up?'

People do mean different things by tiredness. Getting a more thoughtful definition from EB can be a useful filter of the main types of 'tiredness' we see. Lack of motivation and low energy are typical of depression. Weakness and fatigue make me think more of chronic illness, say anaemia. Feeling sleepy in the daytime is often more about sleep apnoea (heavy snoring with periods of complete pauses in breathing during sleep) or even medications that cause drowsiness. And I'd think of chronic fatigue syndrome/myalgic encephalitis (ME) if there was four months or more of physical and mental fatigue that isn't clearly explained by anything else, isn't helped by rest and is linked with a range of other specific symptoms, from muscle pains and headaches to sore throat or memory problems.

'It's weakness really, just fatigue. Like exhaustion. I don't sleep brilliantly, but I wake up feeling OK.'

Fatigue is one of those conditions where it is really important for me to establish the patient's thoughts or concerns early on. In the end, my job with fatigue boils down to three main elements: (1) Make sure it isn't a sign of illness (psychological, physical or both). This might mean investigations as well as listening carefully to the patient's story and an examination. (2) Reassure the patient that everything's normal (if it is) and that he or she will feel better soon. (3) In either case, offer appropriate support through a difficult patch.

But in order to offer meaningful reassurance, I need to know what EB is worried about, if anything.

'And was there anything in particular that you're worried about? Some people have specific worries about what the problem could be – and it's really helpful for me to know if anything's on your mind, however daft you may think it sounds.'

'Umm. Not really. I mean it just doesn't make sense to me, that's all. My wife had an underactive thyroid diagnosed last year, and she was feeling tired a lot – I know that can be a cause for tiredness. I just don't know.'

'Yes, you're right. We certainly need to have thyroid problems on our radar. OK, so can I ask you some rather specific questions then, to rule out a few things?' This is signposting; a courtesy really, showing the patient where I'd like to take the conversation, and asking permission.

'Sure.'

The list of potential causes of fatigue is huge. In fact pretty much any condition could be on it. One of the ironies of a traditional medical education is that we were taught in terms of important diseases rather than common symptoms. So, for example, we'd have lectures on diabetes, arthritis, anaemia or the thyroid, all of which have fatigue as a key feature. But patients don't usually come to the doctor complaining of a disease – they come with symptoms like fatigue, or breathlessness, or painful joints. So for me and my generation of doctors, in effect our learning was a two-step process – step one was to learn all the diseases and their symptoms, and step two involved working out a system for remembering all the diseases that could cause the common symptom the patient in front of us was actually asking us about. Happily, things are changing now – today's medical students are much more likely to have some symptom-based teaching sessions, and modern textbooks often reflect this more practical and patient-centred perspective.

He was right though – where *do* I start? And actually, how long *have* I got? About five minutes now.

(five minutes)

In order to manage this sensibly, I need to call on some old friends. First, the tried and tested history-taking structures I learned at medical school, like a coarse sieve. I need to create a shortlist of possible diagnoses – the so-called 'differential diagnosis' – and then systematically rule some out, or arrange them in a sensible order of likelihood. The diagnostic jargon is 'restricted rule-out' – ruling out conditions from a restricted list of possibles. Then, the need to play safe and rule out any red flags – a much finer sieve. I rely too on my ability to recognise patterns of symptoms in EB's story that could suggest an overarching diagnosis. Finally, there's what you could call clinical intuition, the 'art of general practice': noticing something unusual or which stands out from the expected for this patient. That is one of the great bonuses of knowing the patient well – something which sadly is less common these days as care is increasingly fragmented and shared between doctors. But I'd argue it's still more likely to happen in primary care than in hospital medicine.

'You said stress is not an issue for you at the moment – everything's fine at home and at work – and no problems with your mood at all?'

'No, nothing in that way at all. I'm certainly not depressed or stressed, if that's what you mean.'

'OK, I'm just going through a sort of list at the moment. That's fine.'

I get the sense that he's not a fan of the stress/psychological theories of fatigue. I am not exploring this side of things to piss him off, or to fob him off either. I am exploring it because it is often at the heart of the fatigue we see in general practice. Stressful life events like work problems, family trouble, bereavement or financial difficulties account for about two-thirds of fatigue complaints. I'd be doing him a disservice if I didn't at least explore that possibility.

'And you have had a recent nasty sinusitis, haven't you? Tell me more about all the infections you've been getting.' I'm trying hard to ask open questions – I know they're more fruitful, encouraging EB to tell his story in his own words. But I am not sure how long I'll be able to keep that up. I need to rule out some specifics and I don't have lots of time. I can feel closed, quick-fire questions looming.

A recent illness, typically a viral infection, can certainly cause fatigue for some time after the acute symptoms have passed. EB's sinusitis was particularly severe, now I think back, and he needed strong antibiotics. It wasn't that long ago either. It's possible that it has contributed to his recent fatigue – although on its own it can't really explain symptoms going back for some months. But if he's had several viral infections over the last year – which could just be bad luck – that could easily have given his immune system a knock and left him more susceptible to repeat infections. Admittedly it's a pretty humdrum cause, and I suspect he wouldn't be satisfied with 'repeated viral infections' as an explanation for his fatigue. But it's quite possible. Equally, it's just possible that his immune system is weak for some other reason; for example, a blood disorder like leukaemia or myeloma, making repeated infections more likely. It's much less likely, but I must keep those sort of possibilities at the back of my mind.

'Well, I've had the sinusitis you know about – that was really bad actually. It's still not completely better . . .'

'Yes, and what about the other infections you mentioned . . . I can see a sore throat a few months ago here . . . and a viral infection before that . . . anything else?'

I know this sounds a bit brusque, but I cannot afford to get too distracted from my direction of travel here. If we stopped at every symptom and tried to deal with it, we could be here all day. My priority for him today is to try to make sense of the big picture.

'Um, I just seem to be constantly getting colds, and the sore throat, yes, that has never cleared up really.'

'That is quite a few infections you've had. That, in itself, can knock back your immune system each time you get one, leaving you more prone to future infections, and feeling constantly run down. Let's just keep that in mind, while we think of other possibilities.'

I am deliberately sowing the seeds of possibility here, just making a suggestion that repeated infections could be linked to his exhaustion. I must keep my mind open to other possibilities though, and not close down any diagnostic options prematurely. That's easy to do. It's particularly tempting in clinical exams, when the pressure is on, to make a diagnosis. You make up your mind within the first minute or two that the problem is X, and then direct the patient down an X-shaped consultation, when in fact the problem was Y. You fail.

The joint and muscle aches he briefly mentioned earlier have caught my attention. One possible cause for fatigue is arthritis of various sorts, or the so-called connective tissue disorders. These are auto-immune conditions in which the body's immune system becomes overactive and can start attacking the connective tissues – like joints or muscles or skin. An example is systemic lupus erythematosus (SLE), which can cause joint and muscle pains as well as fatigue. On the other hand, as a fiftyish-year-old man myself, I am acutely aware that muscle and joint aches and niggling pains do start to become everyday companions. And his particular complaint – tennis elbow (or lateral epicondylitis) – is not strictly an arthritic type of problem (inflammation of the joint itself) – it's inflammation of the tendons around the elbow joint, usually caused by repetitive use.

'Tell me more about the muscle and joint problems you mentioned. Apart from the tennis elbow, anything?'

'Well, I had an ankle sprain from cricket last year, and just general niggles, you know. I just seem to be getting lots of aches and strains these days.'

'Any swelling or stiffness of the joints?' I need to get more specific now. Swelling or stiffness of joints would ring more of an alarm bell – cardinal signs of inflammatory arthritis.

'No, I wouldn't say actual swelling, no, just aches and pains.'

'Whereabouts?'

'Well, could be anywhere. My knees can get sore when I've done a long run. The soles of my feet can get sore too . . .'

This is not ringing any major arthritis alarm bells for me. Rheumatoid arthritis, for example, can affect any joint, but typically the first to be affected are the small joints of the hands and feet. This sounds like routine overuse in a middle-aged guy. Plantar fasciitis of the soles of the feet, perhaps some wear and tear of the knee joints. Not typical signs of the connective tissue disorders or the

214

inflammatory arthritides, such as rheumatoid arthritis, that can cause fatigue.

'Do you manage to stay active then? You say you play cricket.'

'Yes, well I'm fairly active, I suppose. I try to go to the gym once a week. But my job does mean I spend a lot of time at my desk.'

'I think that applies to lots of us these days. So, who do you play cricket for then?' I can't resist – and it's good to have some 'human' contact.

'Oh, it's just a wandering side a mate of mine started a few years ago. We're not very good, but it's fun. Do you play?'

'When I can. Not so nimble these days though. I play for my local club occasionally. But I know when I'm not exercising I always start to feel lethargic and tired . . .'

'Yes, you're right there.' I can see him thinking about his own exercise levels and how they might link to his tiredness.

'And are you sleeping OK? You don't wake up early in the morning, for example, and find yourself unable to get back to sleep?'

This can often open the floodgates – lots of us don't sleep the whole way through the night. I slightly wince at myself inside for having asked the question. But I want to make sure he doesn't have obvious insomnia problems, or sleep apnoea. That can make you so tired that you fall asleep during the day – even at the wheel of your car.

'No, I don't wake up early. I sometimes have trouble getting off to sleep though, and I do get up to go to the toilet once in the night, which is annoying.'

Tell me about it – I'm up three or four times at the moment. Self-disclosure by a doctor can be a useful tool, helping to show that one can empathise with a patient's predicament. I might say, for example, 'I've been through something similar, so I'm not at all surprised that you feel that way.' The danger, of course, is that it becomes all about me and my problems. Here, I could easily stray into: 'Oh, I've had that too. It's a real pain, I have to keep getting up in the night . . . etc. etc.' I don't think this is the right moment for self-disclosure.

'Does your wife say you snore?'

'No, not particularly. I probably do, but it's not a problem.'

'But you nap during the day, you said. Do you have any control over that? I mean, do you ever just fall asleep while you're doing something, for example?'

'No. I just feel exhausted and feel the need to go and have a lie-down some days. I never used to have to do that.'

Good. I've managed to avoid opening the floodgates, and that pretty much relegates sleep apnoea, I think, to near the bottom of the list.

(***six minutes***)

'Now, what medications are you taking?'

'Nothing at the moment.'

'And nothing that you buy yourself from the pharmacy or whatever?'

Always worth asking about medications. Fatigue must be almost as common a medication side effect as rashes or diarrhoea.

'No, nothing at all.'

'OK, great. Can I just ask about alcohol?' (We ask everyone this.) 'Do you drink alcohol?'

'Yes.'

Alcohol is a big twenty-first-century problem, particularly binge drinking in bouts. Rates of alcohol-related health problems are soaring, and I need to be alert to the myriad complications too much booze can cause, from brain disorders and neurological problems to abnormal liver blood tests, hepatitis, cirrhosis, liver failure, and even liver cancer. Apart from any of those formal diagnoses, over-drinking can also make some people aggressive; cause accidents; and affect relationships, work performance, mental wellbeing, sleep and energy levels.

'How many units would you say you drink each week? I know it's hard.'

Everyone has to think carefully about this question. Myself included. Until very recently the NHS guidelines were twenty-one

216

units a week for men and fourteen units a week for women. The latest guidance in the UK is that men and women should drink no more than fourteen units of alcohol a week – the equivalent of six pints of average-strength beer or seven glasses of wine – in order to keep their health risks low. Guidelines vary with time and depend on where you are in the world. The UK is now the seventh-strictest EU country in its guidance on alcohol – the Netherlands, Poland and Bulgaria have the tightest limits, and Spain, France and Lithuania are the most relaxed. In the USA men are advised to drink no more than 196 g of ethanol a week, and women no more than 98 g – compared to the UK's new unisex limit of 112 g.

Apart from guidance about them being inconsistent, units of alcohol are not intuitive measures. The number of units in a glass of wine, for example, can range from one or two for a small glass to three or four for one of those massive vases we are often now served in bars and restaurants. The strength of alcoholic drinks can vary enormously too – a pint of strong lager contains three units, whereas a standard-strength lager is just over two. Then there's the problem of estimating a weekly average, when your intake often varies from one week to the next depending on parties, work dos or stress levels. I take people's reports of how much alcohol they drink with a pinch of salt – not because I distrust them, but because I know it's very hard to make a reliable estimate. I've heard people say that doctors automatically double whatever you say, and write that down in the records. I have never heard of that myself, and we certainly don't teach medical students or GP trainees to do that. The doctor–patient relationship has to be built on trust. Having said that, some interesting research has found that the amount of alcohol that we in the UK say we consume only accounts for about 60 per cent of the alcohol that's actually sold. So unless we're chucking 40 per cent of our alcohol away, we are probably all underestimating how much we drink.

Now I need to do a quick 'review of systems' – a run-through of the major bodily systems, focusing on things that might cause fatigue like cancers, diabetes, anaemia, thyroid problems. At the same time, I must make sure I remember to rule out any red flags for fatigue. I focus on EB's bowels (any changes in bowel habit, any blood?); his urinary system (going to the loo often + unusually thirsty = diabetes, any blood in the urine?); and general red flags such as any unintended weight loss (a general red flag for cancer or serious systemic diseases like HIV or TB); any fever, sweats or cough (which could spell malignancy or infections of various sorts)? I check he hasn't travelled anywhere exotic recently.

(*eight minutes*)

All clear.

Now, a couple of questions covering thyroid problems, as that was a particular concern of his.

'Thinking about your thyroid, have you had any unusual hair loss, or noticed that you are more sensitive to the cold or the warm?'

'No – not really. Well, I suppose I do sometimes get a bit sweaty, now I think about it, yes.' The problem with asking leading questions like this is that it can prompt people to promote a barely noticeable, bottom-league-type of symptom straight into the premier division of ailments. I have to listen carefully and make a judgement about how significant the symptom sounds. His hesitation and change in direction makes me question how important this symptom really is. It shouldn't make much difference though – I am thinking we will almost certainly be doing some blood tests, which will cover the main serious causes of sweating I am considering here – thyroid problems, diabetes, infection and malignancy.

'Right, well thanks for that – really helpful. Can I examine you now, please? I'd like to check your lymph nodes, listen to your heart and chest, check your blood pressure and so on?'

As is often the case in general practice, I am aware that my examination is unlikely to prove very fruitful, particularly if no specific conditions have come to light from the patient's history. The real value here is to make sure I haven't missed anything obvious, and to reassure the patient that I have done a thorough check.

I take a general look at him, scanning for the pallor of anaemia, and the subtle yellowing of the eyes or skin in jaundice (often a sign of liver disease). He's fairly skinny. It's very rare, but I'm also keeping an eye out for darkening of his skin – hyperpigmentation can be a sign of Addison's disease, an unusual visitor in primary care, but one that pops its head round the door from time to time. It is a condition in which the adrenal glands don't produce enough of the steroid hormones that they should (like cortisol), which can lead to low blood pressure, muscle aches and pains, and fatigue. It's rare but can be serious if it's not picked up early enough.

I feel for his lymph nodes – in his neck, his armpits, above the collar bone and in his groin. I want to make sure he doesn't have widespread swollen lymph nodes – generalised lymphadenopathy – which can be a sign of generalised infection, some cancers like leukaemia or lymphomas, or even some of the connective tissue disorders. I feel some in his neck but nowhere else. They feel normal size and texture to me – not the firm, hard, painless nodes, often very large, that might make my cancer receptors twitch.

His heart and chest sound normal – always worth a quick listen for any heart failure or signs of chest infection, for example. And I focus particularly on examining his thyroid gland, because he brought it up earlier – although I would check this anyway given his story. This sits at the front of the neck, shaped like a bow tie. I look for any obvious swelling of the gland, and then, standing behind him, gently feel the gland with my fingertips, while explaining that I am not going to strangle him. I am feeling for symmetry, consistency, any masses, and any enlargement. Normal.

I check his blood pressure and feel his pulse (low blood pressure could be due to Addison's disease, for example, and a rapid or irregular pulse might point to a thyroid problem). I quickly examine his abdomen – all reassuringly normal.

(*ten minutes*)

'OK. Well, everything seems to be fine. Your thyroid certainly seems OK when I examine it. And there's nothing to suggest many of the other main causes of fatigue – stress or depression, anaemia, sleep problems, heart or lung trouble, infections or types of arthritis, for example. So that's all very reassuring. At the moment I can't see any obvious patterns that might point to an overarching explanation for all your symptoms either. It is possible that this is all down to a string of infections that have left you struggling – we do see that sometimes. Or a combination of things that on their own aren't significant, but, added together, are taking their toll. And I'll be straight with you and say that we may not be able to put a neat label on it.'

'Mmm. So where do we go from here then? Because I don't feel right at all.'

He's pre-empted me. It's a schoolboy error in medicine, to say that everything's normal. I really mean that all my examining and testing is normal. But of course from the patient's perspective, everything is absolutely not normal. He still feels knackered.

'No, of course. Well I'd suggest we do some blood tests to rule some options out – for example, just to check your thyroid and your sugar levels, and make sure you're not anaemic, that your white blood cells are OK, and that you're not short on any vitamins and so on. Would that be all right?'

'Yes, absolutely, that makes a lot of sense.'

I knew this chap was going to want tests so it was a disingenuous question really. But let me explain my thinking on whether to do any specific tests for this man's fatigue. It's based largely on an excellent article I read in the *British Medical Journal* from a few years back by William Hamilton, a GP and professor of primary care diagnostics, and his colleagues.

For most patients with fatigue, tests are probably not warranted. The research suggests that almost three-quarters of consultations are one-offs – in other words, most people don't come back to see the doctor about their tiredness again. That suggests that most patients' fatigue improves with time, for example as they recover slowly from an infection or the stress in their lives settles down. GPs order tests in only about half of patients with fatigue, and few of these tests come back abnormal. Even so, laboratories are overwhelmed with requests for tests for fatigue because it's such a common symptom. So in an ideal world, rational investigation of fatigue symptoms should avoid unnecessary testing for the majority of patients who don't need it, while at the same time picking up the few patients with an underlying disease without too much delay.

We know that younger patients and patients who consult frequently are less likely to have underlying disease. EB has been quite a few times this year. If there are obvious potential causes for the fatigue, such as a recent infection or stresses, then there's a case for deferring any tests to see if time sorts things out. Time is a useful diagnostic tool. Sometimes, doing nothing is the best option. EB has had several infections, and a severe one fairly recently, which could explain his symptoms. So there are two reasons not to do any tests today, but perhaps to ask him to come back in four weeks if things haven't improved, at which time we could reconsider.

If he had any red-flag symptoms I would also certainly investigate at the first consultation. But he hasn't – no weight loss or fever or widespread lymph node enlargement, and no bowel or urinary red flags either. And for many of the specific conditions I am considering, there's been no clear suggestion of a diagnosis that might tip me into ordering tests – no sleep apnoea, no obvious thyroid problems, no obvious arthritis or connective tissue disorders, no classic symptoms of diabetes. His heart and lungs seem fine.

But with this patient, there's still enough to make me want to do further tests. First, he's mentioned his wife's trouble with her thyroid, and it's hard to rule that out from an examination alone. Sometimes thyroid problems can start subtly. I don't want to look stupid by missing thyroid problems in him when I can easily do the test. Second, although his various symptoms don't clearly add up to any specific diagnosis, there are enough near misses to make me cautious. He also seems very distressed by these symptoms, and he's obviously keen to understand them as much as he can. He's also been to see us several times now, and he's been feeling fatigued for some months already. Without tests, I don't think I am ever likely to satisfy him.

As a doctor it's often hard to resist being thorough – you only remember the ones you miss. Safer to check than to regret not having tested, and risk a complaint or worse.

However there's a question burning in my mind; whether a series of normal results will reassure him, or whether he will just keep on wanting to dig for answers with more and more bizarre tests. It's not uncommon. I am worried that he might do an internet fishing expedition and search for all the possible causes of fatigue, from rare mineral deficiencies to even rarer environmental poisons. And then come and ask me to do the tests. So what's wrong with that? In the words of the patient: where do I start?

Over-testing can be a kind of purgatory for patients, obsessively hunting for more and more obscure causes which simply aren't there. Apart from diverting patients from what may be the real problem – stress, being overweight, inactivity, psychological issues say – if you look hard enough for abnormalities you will find them. The trouble is they are nearly always insignificant abnormalities: a tiny rise in this hormone or that chemical, a miniscule nodule on your lung X-ray, a minor blip on your ECG (heart tracing). All of them probably nothing – but now we, and you, have to do some double-checking to make sure they're *actually* nothing.

All the evidence suggests that for a medical test to have any real value, there needs to be a reasonable chance that something's wrong in that area in the first place. It's what's called the pre-test probability. If you give someone a chest X-ray because they have the signs and symptoms of a chest infection, then any abnormality or shadow is useful information – it's highly likely to represent something significant. But if you just do a chest X-ray on someone without any symptoms, any abnormalities that show up are more likely to be meaningless noise. But once you've found that little nodule on a lung, you might need to do another chest X-ray or a CT scan or a bronchoscopy – all very expensive procedures, some with real risks to your health, not to mention the inconvenience and worry. That's the danger of blind fishing expeditions – just testing for every possible cause – and why a rational approach means testing based on the history and examination.

For fatigue, the evidence suggests that an initial screen should include tests for only the commonest diagnoses. That's checking haemoglobin (anaemia), the erythrocyte sedimentation rate (ESR – a general measure of inflammation, which might flag up arthritis or a cancer, for example), glucose (diabetes), and thyroid tests. Liver function and kidney function tests might be particularly useful in older patents or where there are specific concerns about kidneys or liver (say itching or alcohol problems). Some guidelines recommend checking for coeliac disease too – a sensitivity to gluten which can affect the absorption of vitamins and minerals from the gut.

More specialised checks might include for glandular fever in a younger person with fatigue and swollen lymph nodes and a sore throat – but it's unlikely in Mr EB. I might also check Vitamin D if someone was at risk of deficiency because they were housebound, used sunscreens regularly, had darker skin (for example, if they were of African, African-Caribbean, or South Asian origin), or had reduced gut absorption. I might even think about HIV or hepatitis testing, if they were at risk, or a chest X-ray if I was worried about TB, for example. If someone had the relevant history or findings on examination, I might check for much rarer conditions – for example, if they had a rash and a history of tick bites I would check for Lyme disease. A specific test for iron can be sensible in women of childbearing age.

I'm tired now and I think there's every chance that Mr EB will be back again and again if we don't do a big battery of tests now. He has struggled with tiredness for three months or more already. Why waste his time and ours by making him come back again later if all the first-line tests are normal?

I type in my full battery of tests for TATT – all the usual first-line ones, but with a few extras like Vitamin B12 and Vitamin D thrown in for good measure. I know it's not exactly evidence-based, but I suspect playing by the rule book in this case might be a false economy.

'There you go – all in the computer. So, if you make an appointment for those tests, and then ring up a few days afterwards for the results. Then perhaps if all is normal – which I suspect will be the case – leave it a month or so to see if things improve for you. And if you're still struggling, then come back to see me and we can look at you again. How does that sound?'

'OK, I'll do the blood tests and see how it goes. And what about my sinuses and sore throat . . .?'

'I think they really should gradually improve over that period. If not, we'll discuss them next time. If they're any worse in the meantime, come back sooner of course. OK?'

I stand up and offer my hand for a goodbye shake.

'OK, thanks, Doctor. Door open or closed?'

'Oh open, thanks.' Always open.

(*twelve minutes*)

Chapter 13

Mrs CH

(running thirty-one minutes late)

Doctor view

Appointment time: 9.30
Name: Mrs CH
Age: 35 years old
Occupation: Housewife and mother
Past medical history:
Two uncomplicated pregnancies
Medication:
Levothyroxine 50 mcg
Reminders:
Cervical smear due in three months
Last consultation:
Saw me two months ago when we started her on levothyroxine – synthetic thyroid hormone – for her underactive thyroid gland. She has recently had blood tests to check how she is responding to her new medication.

Patient view

Mrs CH has been feeling generally tired for the last six months or so, with slightly heavier periods and some weight gain. She made an appointment to see the doctor about three months ago because she had developed some tingling in her hands and fingers, especially at night. The doctor examined her and arranged some blood tests, which were all normal except for an underactive thyroid gland (hypothyroidism).

She was relieved to have a diagnosis, and in a way not surprised to hear it was her thyroid, as her mother had an underactive thyroid too. Since starting the thyroid pills two months ago, she has been feeling a lot better, with more energy. Her periods are not quite back to normal yet, and she's still a little overweight, but the tingling in her hands has stopped.

She's back today for a routine follow-up review, which the doctor asked her to book last time.

'Hello, I'm so sorry to keep you waiting . . .'

'Don't worry, I'm not in a rush. I expect you're very busy, aren't you?'

Mrs CH is a lovely lady – for two reasons. First, she is actually lovely – thoughtful, polite, always smiling (if there are two types of people in life, energy boosters and energy sappers, she is definitely a booster). But second, she seems particularly lovely to me today because I think she is bringing good news and might even let me catch up on time. The irony is that I would love to spend more time chatting to her, wallowing in her positivity and my diagnostic and therapeutic glory. But when you're up against the clock you can't dwell too long on your successes, and, as in much of life, it's often the least demanding people who get the least attention.

I am feeling optimistic because I have already had a peek at her blood results. Two months after starting treatment with levothyroxine (replacement thyroid hormone) for her underactive thyroid, her blood test levels are now in the normal range. I'm not jumping to any conclusions though – it's the person, not her biochemistry that I'm really interested in. When it comes to the thyroid, what the blood tests say and what the patient says don't always tally.

For such a tiny gland, the thyroid can cause a hell of a lot of problems. If you think of the cells and tissues of your body as an orchestra, then your thyroid is the conductor. It keeps your body functioning at a nice steady rhythm. It works by producing a hormone called thyroxine, which is carried round the body in the bloodstream.

When the thyroid is not working hard enough, the body orchestra plays to a slower beat. An underactive thyroid gland (hypothyroidism) can cause all sorts of symptoms, ranging from fatigue and weight gain to skin changes and depression. There are so many possible symptoms linked to hypothyroidism, most of them not specific to thyroid disease, that diagnosing it can sometimes drag on. It's also common for people not to have any symptoms to speak of at all.

Three months ago, when Mrs CH mentioned changes to her menstrual periods, and carpal tunnel syndrome (a condition in which a nerve in your wrist comes under pressure, causing pain, tingling or weakness, mainly in your forearm and hand), my thyroid warning system switched to alert mode. Together, we built a picture of several vaguely thyroid-shaped problems that had been going on a while, from fatigue to weight gain and even a suggestion of intolerance of the cold, which prompted me to check her thyroid hormone levels. They showed a clear-cut underactive thyroid, and we decided to start her on the usual treatment, levothyroxine (a synthetic version of thyroxine, also called T4, the thyroid hormone). I plumped for a low starting dose of 50 micrograms. I know she's chemically back to normal; today we'll see if she feels any better in herself.

'So, how are you feeling?' I say, with the look of a hopeful father asking about a day of school exams.

'Well, much better actually, thank you, Doctor. *Much* more energy, and just generally better. I can't say I've lost much weight to speak of, unfortunately, but the tingling's gone now.' She looks down at her hands, opening and closing them.

'Oh, that's great news. And what about periods – any improvement?'

'No, not really – not yet anyway.'

'Well, that may take a little while to settle down. And are you having any side effects or problems with the thyroxine tablets?'

'No, I don't think so, nothing really.'

'Great, great. Well look, the blood tests do show that things are pretty much back to normal now, which is excellent.' I invite her to look at the computer screen.

(**two minutes**)

'So, we measure two main hormones to check the thyroid . . .'

The bland numbers on the screen belie the staggering beauty of the thyroid hormone system behind them. It's such a clever, delicately choreographed dance – and it's just one small sideshow in a grand hormonal ballet.

The thyroid gland is shaped like a bow tie and sits in your neck, in front of your windpipe. It's only about 2–3 cm across. It makes, and then pumps out, thyroxine into your bloodstream. The really clever bit is how the body monitors levels of thyroxine in the blood, and then adjusts how much the thyroid makes. The master monitoring centre is the pea-sized pituitary gland, sitting at the base of your brain behind the bridge of your nose. It can sense the tiniest of fluctuations in levels of thyroxine in the bloodstream. When it senses too little, it pumps out more of a hormone that drives the thyroid gland to work harder and make more thyroxine (called thyroid-stimulating hormone, or TSH for short). It's a feedback loop; one of many the body relies on.

'So when I am trying to make sense of your thyroid blood tests,' I say, drawing a rough circular diagram of a thyroid feedback loop, 'I need to know the levels of both thyroxine (the main thyroid hormone), and TSH (the hormone which drives the thyroid). When you had your first tests, your T4 (thyroid hormone) level – here – was well below the normal range, and your TSH – this one – was well above its normal level. That combination – low levels of thyroid hormone, and high levels of the TSH hormone that's trying to drive the thyroid gland to make more – is the biochemical signature of an underactive thyroid gland.'

So far, my thyroid testing explanation is a bit like a nuclear physicist comparing atoms with snooker balls – it's OK for getting the general idea, but in reality things are much more complex and mysterious. Fortunately Mrs CH is happy with snooker balls. She's feeling much better. But in my experience patients don't always feel as well as they would like, and snooker balls aren't always enough. We'd all love the science to give us clear guidance – but sometimes, and thyroid treatment is a good example, our decisions have to much more nuanced.

For a start, there are times when the patient's blood tests and symptoms don't seem to tally. This can cause confusion and frustration for both patients and doctors. The first problem is when you don't have symptoms but your TSH is high (suggesting an underactive thyroid) and levels of thyroxine, the thyroid hormone, are normal. This means you're making enough thyroxine, but the thyroid gland needs extra stimulation from the TSH to keep up. There are two main options in this case: the first is simply to monitor your levels closely and treat when they hit a threshold or you develop symptoms, and the second, for certain groups, is to start a trial of treatment anyway. Thyroid experts differ in their favoured approach, and often it comes down to individual circumstances. The other issue is when patients are being treated for an underactive thyroid, and their blood tests suggest they are back in normal thyroid territory, but they don't feel like they are. Then we can get into discussions, sometimes lively, about the pros and cons of upping the dose of thyroxine even though the levels are normal. It's well recognised that some people do feel healthier when their thyroxine replacement dose is tending towards over-treatment, and sometimes I'm open to that idea. But if I'm reluctant, it's because I know that long-term over-treatment with thyroid hormone can cause heart problems and bone thinning. 'First do no harm' is reverberating around my skull.

Last, but by no means least, is my terror of T3. T3 is the active form of the thyroid hormone in the body. Except in rare cases, if you have enough T4 (thyroxine), your body will naturally convert it to T3. But some people who don't feel wholly better on the usual thyroxine (T4) treatment, and who have researched all this in detail, wonder about adding T3 to their treatment. Some people want to try a natural thyroid extract, for example, which contains both T3 and T4. I'm sometimes presented with printouts from a website or even research papers backing up a request for me to prescribe it. But however much I might want to give them what they want, I have to be guided by the current medical consensus, based on appraisal of all the medical literature. That can be really frustrating for patients, and often for me too. New research findings can take ages to translate into changes in clinical practice; on average about seventeen years. But it's right that before treatments are rolled out they are tested thoroughly to make sure they are safe and effective. At the moment, the expert advice is that there isn't enough evidence to suggest that combinations of T4 and T3 offer any advantage over standard T4 therapy on its own. And there are safety concerns; one is that T3 is five times more active than T4 so there is a risk of over-treatment if the dose of T3 is not carefully controlled. As the experts remind me, I have a professional responsibility not to prescribe any potentially harmful therapies without proven advantages over the existing treatments. But perhaps more pertinent for a busy generalist, at the moment the advice from medically qualified thyroid specialists is that the addition of T3 in any form is not normally recommended. Some specialists might feel comfortable giving it a go, but it's a brave generalist who swims against that tide.

Anyway, I'm hugely relieved that we seem to have side-stepped any of those conundrums today.

'So you seem to be feeling better, and your thyroid tests are back to normal. I'd suggest carrying on with the same dose and checking the bloods again in three months? What do you think?'

'Yes, that sounds good. So, I'll make an appointment for the blood test nearer the time, shall I?'

'Yes, at reception. You don't need to fast before that one. And, of course, you must let us know if any of the symptoms are returning, or you feel unwell at any time.'

'Yes, of course, Doctor, thank you so much.'

'It's a pleasure. Good to see you.'

I show her to the door. I sit back down and type up the notes:

'Patient reviewed. Feels much better on 50 micrograms levothyroxine. More energy, less fatigued. Tingling in fingers resolved completely. Little change to weight or periods yet.

'TSH: 0.4, T4: 14. No side effects reported. O/E Pulse 70/min and regular. No thyroid swelling or other signs. Continue at current dosage and review in six months with results of thyroid function tests. Sooner if problems.'

(*five minutes*)

Mrs CH really has been an energy boost. We spotted her problem, and made a difference to her life. She said thank you. And it only took five minutes.

Short consultations are a breath of fresh air. But they are few and far between: the odd patient coming back to say all is well perhaps, contraceptive pill checks, single minor illness worries (rare), requests for repeat prescriptions or sick notes; those are the main ones. For all the others, ten minutes just seems inadequate. Too often it feels as if I am fire-fighting. And probably because appointments are so difficult to come by, and they're only ten minutes long, patients will try to squeeze in more than one problem. It's annoying – but I don't really blame them.

GPs' workloads are ballooning, and many say they are at breaking point. One estimate suggests that the clinical workload in UK general practice has increased by about 40 per cent since 1998. This is mostly down to an ageing population – we're seeing a significant rise in the number of consultations with people over the age of sixty. At the same time, as the population ages, so does the number of patients with at least one long-term condition, making consultations more complex and time-consuming. We spend much more time nowadays on preventing illness, too – for example, checking blood pressures and cholesterol levels, monitoring long-term chronic conditions, doing health checks or writing care plans. We try to involve patients more in decisions about their care – which is welcome progress, but it all takes time. Changes to the way GP practices are monitored and paid mean more administrative box-ticking and, since 2012, GPs have also been asked to take the lead in commissioning health services for the NHS – diverting many from their frontline clinical work towards working for local Clinical Commissioning Groups.

Patients are seeing their GP more often, too. In the UK in the last decade the average number of times a patient visits their family physician each year has almost doubled from three to nearly six times a year, with the elderly consulting up to fourteen times a year. The European average is six times a year, ranging from an average twelve visits a year in Hungary to three visits per year in Sweden (this is possibly because Sweden has many nurses delivering primary care). But most European countries have seen increases in consultation rates with primary care doctors in the last ten years; the same is true in the United States because of dwindling numbers of family physicians. So those intimate minutes with the doctor are extremely precious, and as people live longer and medicine can do more and more, there's more than ever to cram in.

At the same time, the GP workforce is changing and resources have not kept pace with demand. The Royal College of General Practitioners (RCGP) estimates that we are about 10,000 GPs short in the UK. Many experienced GPs are nearing retirement or opting to take early retirement, more and more GPs work part-time (partly due to increasing 'feminisation' of the GP workforce), and in many parts of the country recruitment to GP posts is a struggle.

Consultation times are expanding in a desperate attempt to squeeze in more and more. But it's still not enough. In the past thirty years, consultation times in the UK have roughly doubled. From six to seven minutes in the 1970s and 1980s, the average consultation expanded to 8.33 minutes in 1990, and was 9.36 minutes by 1997. The most up-to-date figures suggest that the average length of time for a surgery consultation with a GP partner in 2006/7 was 11.7 minutes, shorter than in many other developed countries. (Whenever I can, I now do a mix of ten- and fifteen-minute appointments; it avoids the built-in wait for patients and cuts stress levels for this doctor.)

Inconveniently for the fifteen-minute-appointment lobbyists like me, the research evidence in favour of increasing consultation times is mixed. Lots of studies have shown an association between consultation length and markers of consultation quality, such as patients feeling more empowered to take control of their care. But a high-quality review of several studies some years ago concluded that there was insufficient evidence from controlled trials (the scientific gold standard of evidence) to conclude that longer consultations improve outcomes for patients or patient satisfaction. However, a more recent review did indicate a likely benefit of longer consultations for patients with psychological problems. There's also some evidence that longer consultations mean fewer return consultations for the same problem.

Some doctors still take enormous pride in their ability to plough through huge lists of patients like a pack of cards. Good for them – in some ways I admire their express consulting skills. But I don't think we should settle for the 'stack 'em high and sell 'em cheap' approach to medicine; it short-changes us and our patients, and it's not the sort of care I'd want to give a relative of mine. Nor is it what I was trained for. Ten minutes is just too short to combine a modern patient-centred approach to gathering information, doing a careful examination, and involving patients in making management plans. It takes several minutes for an elderly patient just to get to my room and undress for an examination, for goodness' sake. As the RCGP and other professional groups argue, longer consultations of at least fifteen minutes need to become the norm, with flexibility for changing patient needs. That probably means more funding for primary care, and more doctors. We just need time for caring.

Chapter 14

Mr DG

*(**running twenty-six minutes late**)*

Doctor view

Appointment time: 9.40
Name: Mr DG
Age: 73 years old
Occupation: Retired pilot
Past medical history:
  Hypertension
  High cholesterol
  Low Vitamin D
  Migraine
  Chronic obstructive pulmonary disease
  (COPD)
Medication:
  Amlodipine (for blood pressure)
  Seretide inhaler (for COPD)
  Sumatriptan (for migraines)
  Simvastatin (for cholesterol)
Reminders:
  COPD review due
  Blood pressure check required
Last consultation:
  Routine blood tests last week with
  healthcare assistant. No particular
  symptoms mentioned. PSA test added
  at patient's request.

Patient view

Mr DG has to have his blood tests and blood pressure checked once a year as a routine monitor of his health and medication. He came to the surgery a week ago for the tests, and asked for a PSA (prostate cancer blood test) as he hadn't had one for several years. He was completely well and didn't mention any symptoms. When he rang the surgery for his results, the receptionist passed on the message that his PSA level was high and he should make an appointment to discuss this with the doctor.

He has talked this over briefly with his wife and his best friend at the golf club, who knows someone with prostate cancer. Naturally he's concerned that something may be wrong, but he understands that the test is not perfect, so he is not too worried about the request to discuss this with the doctor, with whom he gets on very well.

There's something unnerving about hearing bad news about someone's health before they do. It's uninvited intelligence and brings a guilty burden. In the next ten minutes my task is to lob a hefty black rock into the still, bright water of Mr DG's world.

On recent visits he has kept me updated on his new grandchildren, who he adores, and we've laughed about our golfing disasters. I've quizzed him about what it was like to fly a jumbo-jet; I'm impressed by the skill and the responsibility involved. One summer a few years ago I saw him at home when he had a head-splitting migraine that he thought might be a stroke. I remember his beaming wife, the kitchen coffee smells, family photos in the hall, and his garden bursting with colour and care.

His PSA test result is through the roof: 105 ng/ml. For someone his age, over seventy, anything higher than about 5 ng/ml is considered outside the normal range in our part of the world. PSA stands for prostate-specific antigen. The PSA test is a blood test that measures the level of PSA in your blood. PSA is a protein made by the prostate gland, and some of it naturally leaks into a man's bloodstream – how much depends on your age and the health and size of your prostate. A raised level can mean you have prostate cancer, but it doesn't automatically spell bad news; the test is far from foolproof. Lots of other non-cancer problems can cause a slightly raised PSA test result, from an enlarged prostate (very common as men get older) or inflammation of the prostate (prostatitis) to urine infections or even having recently ejaculated. So I can often reassure men with a mildly raised PSA that it's unlikely to be cancer. But once you're up in the hundreds, reassurance is harder. It becomes much more likely that it really is prostate cancer (some estimates suggest up to a 90 per cent chance at that level). So, for him, this is likely to mean seeing a specialist for further testing at the very least (including a biopsy of the prostate), a high chance of a cancer diagnosis, and lots of talk about radiotherapy, chemotherapy or hormone therapy, and the worry that comes with that.

I need to use some of the time I won back in the last appointment to prepare. A lot hinges on the next few minutes. It's a one-off chance to make a real difference for DG. If I get it right it can make whatever he and his family might face clearer, more bearable, and less frightening. It sets the tone for our future relationship, too. Get it wrong, and they could spend the next few weeks or months confused, frightened, untrusting or even angry.

I recheck the result. Yes, definitely 105 ng/ml. I check the normal range for our local laboratory. I know these numbers, but I want to make sure there hasn't been an obvious error here. I need to be very clear on how we'll manage this too. DG is likely to ask about his options, what will happen next and so on. I need to have that information at my fingertips. I scan the Clinical Knowledge Summaries (CKS) website page about raised PSA tests – a useful evidence-based summary for a busy GP. I double-check the local guidelines for urgent (to be seen within two weeks) referrals for suspected prostate cancer. I know these too, but I want to see what other information might be needed when I send the referral form. The general advice on the form is to refer anyone with a PSA level above their age-specific range, measured on two occasions four weeks apart. But for someone with a PSA level above 20, it says to refer immediately. Check. It also suggests that I should do a urine test to rule out any infection or blood in the urine. And order a blood test to check his kidney function, mainly in case he needs a special contrast scan, which can be affected by poorly functioning kidneys.

I'm wondering whether I should do a digital rectal examination of DG's prostate, too. In other words, put a finger up his bottom to feel the smooth walnut-sized prostate gland. I would certainly do this if someone had a mildly raised PSA – any firm nodules, hardness or asymmetry would increase my suspicion of cancer. But I know he will need to be referred to the specialists anyway for further testing, and they are almost certain to do one themselves. No one needs two fingers up their bottom when one will do, particularly when they've just been on the sharp end of some bad news.

I also need a rapid refresher on my communication skills – the 'breaking bad' variety. A full-time GP might have to break bad news (or 'difficult' news, as it is now described – what I might class as 'bad', the patient might see more positively) about once or twice a month. It isn't always cancer though – it's equally tough to hear you have diabetes for example, or chronic obstructive pulmonary disease, or a positive HIV result. Often I have to break 'probably bad' news – I can't be 100 per cent certain it's cancer yet because you need further tests for which I'm about to refer you, but I'm pretty sure it is. In those situations – like Mr DG's – it's usually best to shoot straight. Most people would rather know of my suspicions, and they often have a pretty good idea themselves anyway. Much worse to go for further tests, blissfully ignorant of any possible gloom, and then suddenly hear that it's cancer. Then the patient is dumped into an unexpected nightmare, and I look like a clueless quack because I didn't mention I had an inkling. I have trained medical students and GP trainees in how to break bad news. But whether it's 'bad', 'probably bad', or 'difficult', it's rarely an easy conversation. It's always worth spending even a minute thinking through how those crucial soft skills might apply in this particular situation.

When I was more junior I learned a lot about breaking bad news from my consultants – often, how not to do it. There was the odd one who would sweep from bed to bed, announcing death sentences as if they were telling the patient what was for lunch. Nurses would be desperately trying to whip a curtain round the bed before the bombshell was actually dropped. Then they'd be left to clear up the debris, with the patient sniffling as the team flew on to the next pyjama'd target. Maybe they had their reasons – studies have found that doctors struggle to break bad news sensitively when they are burned out, fatigued, facing personal difficulties, or have subjective attitudes that could influence their behaviour, such as a personal fear of death. But it felt wrong, and it was upsetting to see our role models behaving in such an inhumane way.

Nowadays learning the skills of breaking bad news is part of the core curriculum at medical school. But back then it was a revelation to have a whole teaching session dedicated to it, with one of the world's recognised experts on bereavement, psychiatrist Colin Murray-Parks. I remember it as one of the great highlights of my five years at medical school. Some of my more scientifically minded friends probably sniggered at it from the back row, but for me these human skills seemed to fill a gaping hole in a course designed to prepare me for caring for humans. We'd learn, for example, about the importance of making sure the environment was right – not too noisy, not in the middle of a corridor, no phones or bleeps going off. There is no one-size-fits-all approach. The key is to clarify what the individual patient already knows; about any tests, or the diagnosis or the condition. Patients often have an inkling that something isn't right – it can be a huge relief to realise they are already half the way there. There's no point launching into a discussion about stuff they already know, either. Do they have any particular concerns or expectations about what is going to happen, and does the family have any queries? It's often helpful to give people a warning shot near the start: 'I'm afraid I have some bad news . . .' Or, 'I'm afraid the tests are not what we had hoped.' That allows people mentally to prepare a little for what's to come. Use clear language, avoid jargon. And, as always, when you're giving information, give it in small chunks and check the patient has understood ('chunk and check'). We know from studies – and experience – that after you've heard some bad news, you don't tend to remember much else of what was said.

Breaking bad news is a complex skill – not only do you have to know your stuff and choose your words thoughtfully, you also have to be tuned in to the patient's non-verbal messages and emotions. You have to react to how people are reacting. Then you have to gauge how much the patient wants to know and be honest, while keeping some hope alive when there may be very little. Sometimes it helps me to have some sort of map or *aide-mémoire* to remind me where I'm going in this sort of consultation. I need to treat my MAD – my Medical Acronym Deficiency. I have a quick glance on the web at one of my favourites – the SPIKES model of breaking bad news, which has six key steps: **S**etting up the interview (including the physical environment, and building rapport with the patient), then assessing the patient's **P**erception (What do they know? Do they have any worries? And so on . . .); obtaining the patient's **I**nvitation (many patients may not want to know everything about the condition or their prognosis – it's a valid psychological coping mechanism); giving **K**nowledge and information to the patient (keep it simple, 'chunk and check'); addressing the patient's **E**motions with **E**mpathetic response; and having a **S**trategy and **S**ummarising (involving the patient in any plans).

I know all of this, but it reminds me to ask DG about what he knows already before I launch into anything. I take my phone off the hook, arrange the chair so we're facing each other without being 'in your face', and print out some patient information leaflets about the PSA test and prostate cancer. So now I'm feeling a bit like I imagine a trapeze artist feels as they do their long warm-up swings before an elaborate fly-and-catch routine: well drilled but aware there's plenty of scope for letting my partner down, and sending them tumbling to the safety-net below.

(*four minutes*)

'Mr DG? Hello, good to see you, come through . . .' We already have a good rapport. I am glad to see him, and glad that it is me who has to tell him.

'You've come about the blood test results, is that right?' I don't want to assume anything here – it's easy to end up several minutes into the consultation talking at crossed purposes.

'Yes, that's right; they told me the old prostate test was high and to come and see you.' That's a relief; we're on the same page and he knows it's about his prostate. My concern is that his face is open and unconcerned. He's verging on jolly.

'So, before we discuss the results, can you just fill me in – what was the thinking behind doing the test? Did you have any urinary symptoms, for example?'

'No, not really. All well in that department. It was just that I hadn't had one for a few years, and you know, they say someone of my age ought to get his prostate checked every so often. So I asked for it to be added on to my usual tests for the blood pressure and so on.'

'And do you know much about the test? How good a test it is, for example, and what it tests for?'

'Well it's for prostate cancer, isn't it? I know it's not 100 per cent as a test – one of my golf friends had it recently actually – it was high but in the end everything was fine after they did more tests. So I know it isn't perfect – I think you gave me a leaflet about it a few years ago actually.'

I'm glad he understands that it's not a perfect test for prostate cancer. That is why we don't see it as a routine test for men without symptoms, and why the NHS in the UK doesn't have a national screening programme for prostate cancer at the moment. In some countries men over fifty are encouraged to have their PSA checked every year; in the UK, the government feels that the evidence has not yet proven that the benefits would outweigh the risks. In the meantime, the national policy here is that we're happy to do the test if a man over fifty wants one, but we usually give him a leaflet first which explains the pros and cons of having the test when you don't have any particular symptoms. I was involved in developing the original leaflet for the health service, so I have rehearsed the arguments and sifted the evidence many times. And argument is the right word – PSA testing is controversial and emotions often run high.

It seems intuitively sensible to have the test – better to be safe than sorry. The logic behind a patient's request for a PSA test is often that a simple blood test could catch the disease early while it's still treatable. It could, and for some men it does. The snag is that, so far, we don't have bulletproof evidence from trials that screening the whole population of healthy men for prostate cancer saves more lives, and testing men without any symptoms may actually do more harm than good. One European study has shown that deaths from prostate cancer could be reduced by 20 per cent if there was a screening programme, but also found that lots of men were being diagnosed and treated unnecessarily. Between thirty-three and forty-eight men would need to be diagnosed and treated to save the life of one man over a ten-year period. But another big American study of prostate cancer screening found no significant reduction in the number of deaths.

The core of the problem is that the PSA test is far from perfect. It has high false positive and false negative rates: in other words, roughly two out of three men with a raised PSA will not have prostate cancer (false positive), and it can miss some men (as many as one in five) who later turn out to have prostate cancer (false negative). Researchers are busy trying to develop a more accurate version of the PSA test, for example by looking at how PSA levels change over time, and comparing the PSA level to prostate size. But until those tests are widely available, we have to make decisions based on a flawed measure.

Abnormal results – which may or may not mean cancer – can lead to unnecessary anxiety and painful diagnostic biopsies (where tissue samples are taken from the prostate to confirm or exclude the diagnosis – though even these aren't perfect either), which can cause bleeding and infection. Even if the tests do then pick up an early prostate cancer, it can sometimes be hard to know whether it will be slow-growing or more aggressive – whether it will behave like a pussy cat or a tiger. From post-mortem examination studies the old medical adage still holds true; most men tend to die *with* the disease rather than *from* it. So some men will end up having unnecessary treatments such as surgery or radiotherapy for a cancer that never would have shortened their life or caused them any problems. The side effects of treatment aren't trivial either: they can cause long-term urinary problems (including incontinence), diarrhoea, infertility and sexual dysfunction.

Of course, for some men, a true negative test will provide welcome reassurance that all is well. And for those men who have a true positive, they may benefit from having an aggressive cancer picked up early and treated. But while those men may benefit, many others may suffer significant harm from having the test. That is why, as a doctor, I feel obliged to explain the situation as honestly as possible *before* a man has the test. It is hugely complicated and the evidence is bewildering and conflicting. I'm not surprised that after I've tried to explain it all, some patients just want me to tell them what to do: 'But what would you do, Doctor?' I stand my ground – I really think this is one of the areas where it has to be the patient's decision. I wouldn't recommend a PSA test for a man without symptoms any more than I would recommend him a partner; it all depends on your personal values, your attitude to life and risk. I've known several people to profoundly regret ever having asked for the test because of the convoluted, anxious and unnecessary journey it has set them on. Others would rather take the test, however uncertain and whatever the costs. Sometimes I attempt to summarise the pros and cons by saying to the patient something like: 'On the one hand it may pick up cancer early when it can still be treated; and a normal result could put your mind at rest. On the other hand, it is not a very accurate test for prostate cancer, and could lead to unnecessary worry or further invasive medical tests and even surgery with unpleasant side effects that you don't actually need.'

'Yes, you're right,' I say, 'it's far from perfect. Lots of things that aren't cancer can cause a raised PSA result – infections, inflammation of the prostate, even ejaculation. But the higher the result is, the more likely it is to be a cancer.'

'I see. So what was my result, Doctor?'

'Now, I'm afraid to say it's not good news.' I'm looking into his eyes, and I can feel a hint of a frown. 'The result is much higher than we'd like. The normal range for someone of your age is up to about 5. Your reading was 105.' I stop to let that sink in, and give him space to reflect and react.

'Right.' He's doing an internal search now, staring down and off to the left in the mid-distance. He's an intelligent man. I guess he's thinking about what this means for him, his wife, his family. 'I see. So what exactly does that mean then?'

'Well, as I say, we can often put a slightly raised test result down to the less serious stuff. But the higher it gets, the more likely it is actually a prostate cancer. And at this level – 105 – I'm afraid there is a pretty good chance that this does mean you have prostate cancer.'

I don't want to leave it there – he needs to understand that (a) although it's highly likely, this is not yet a watertight diagnosis and (b) even if it is prostate cancer, we don't know whether it's a pussy cat or a tiger, whether it's spread, and how it might respond to treatment.

'Now, having said that, we can't be *absolutely* certain without doing further tests. And even if it is cancer, some are very slow-growing and may never cause you serious problems.' I am trying to offer some hope here, at the same time as painting him a realistic picture. I don't like seeing someone upset any more than the next person does, but I see my twin duties here as honesty and compassion.

'Right, I see . . . So . . . OK . . . There we are then.' This sort of speech turbulence is typical of someone doing some internal struggling. Emotions are spilling out into his speech; he can't speak fluently at the moment. It's a cue that is sometimes worth picking up on. I leave some silent space deliberately, and then . . .

'This sort of news can take a while to sink in.'

'Yes. Sorry, Doc, I'm just sort of getting my head round it, you know.'

'Of course. No problem. You take your time. Did you want to ask me anything?'

'Yes, I suppose so. I mean, what do we do now? More tests, is it?'

'Yes, you will need a biopsy of the prostate gland – a small procedure to take a sample of tissue from the gland – that is how we make a firm diagnosis. And that needs to be done in hospital by the specialist team of urologists. So the next step would be a referral to them.'

I deliberately check myself. He seems a bit shell-shocked. He's probably only taking in a small percentage of what I'm saying.

'Right, and will that happen soon, do you think, or is it a long wait?'

'Well, the good news is that you can see them very quickly, within two weeks certainly.' It's great to be able to say that with confidence. It wasn't that long ago that it was a bit of a lottery.

'OK, and where would that be then?'

'Do you have any preferences? We're lucky here, we've got about four different hospitals, all of them very good, where you can choose to go for this sort of referral. Do you have a preference?'

I show him the list of four. He has a careful think and chooses a close one that he likes. It's nice to involve him in a decision – realistically he doesn't have much choice over what happens next, but at least he can choose where it happens. We're in comfortable territory here, a focused task, choosing from a menu. It's a bit of light relief from an intense conversation.

'Right, well I can sort that out today and you should hear about an appointment within the next few days. If you haven't heard within a week, you must let me know. OK?'

'OK, thanks, Doc.'

(*eight minutes*)

There's a silence, as DG thinks. This is a rare moment when the computer can be a useful communication prop. I want to let him think without staring at him while he does it.

'OK, well let me write a few notes down in the computer then. While I do that, I'll let you have a little think about things, and any questions or queries you might have. OK?'

'Sure, go ahead.'

I am filling out the proforma for an urgent suspected urological cancer two-week referral. It reminds me to check his kidney function and get a urine sample. Breaking bad news is a crucial communication task but I don't want to forget my basic medical duties in the process.

I feel the need to acknowledge the emotional burden of what I've just dumped on him. It's in my SPIKES acronym, but I am not just checking off a tick-list here. We don't have a touchy-feely kind of relationship normally, but I think it is important at least to acknowledge the impact this may have on him and his family, and give him the chance to open up a bit, now or later, if he wants to. But I need to choose my words so they don't sound too saccharine. They need to be authentic; reflect the real nature of our relationship.

'I imagine it's not easy hearing this sort of news, is it?'

'No, it certainly isn't, Doc,' he says with a laughy snort. I stay silent, smiling.

'I'm not going to enjoy telling the wife, that's for sure.'

'No, of course. How do you think she'll take it?'

'Well, it's hard to say. She'll just want what's best for me – she'll support me. I just don't want her to worry about it unnecessarily, that's all.' It's good to bring his wife into the consultation, even though she isn't actually in the room.

'Absolutely. Well, is there anything I can do to help with that? Maybe give you some information to take home about the test and what happens next, or talk to her perhaps, on the phone?'

'Information would be good – thanks, Doc, that would be useful I think. She may want to talk to you. Can we keep that up our sleeve?'

'Of course. And you can ring us if you think of any questions or worries after you get home – that's often when they hit you. I can't promise we'll answer there and then – but we'll always be happy to ring you back.'

'Thank you, that's good to know.' Then, after a gap: 'But you think it's pretty much definitely cancer then, do you?'

'I'm afraid I think it's very likely, yes.'

Stop there. Stick with a short clear message. We have already discussed the uncertainty and the small possibility of it not being a serious problem for him.

'And if it is cancer, what can be done about it?'

'Well, there are several likely options – things like radiotherapy, chemotherapy or hormone therapy. They are effective treatments – how effective depends on the type of cancer and how far advanced it is. They do have some potential side effects. I don't want to burden you with lots of details about that right now, but it is all in this leaflet, and I'll be happy to talk through any queries you have.'

'OK. Thanks, Doc. Well, let's get these other tests done then; the sooner the better, I suppose.'

'Yes, right you are. I'll fax that referral off right away. Now, can I just ask for two more routine things? I need a urine sample and a blood test for your kidneys. Here's a pot for the urine – just hand it in at reception if you can manage a sample right now – can you?'

'I'm not sure – I'll have a go.'

'Well, if you can. And if you could ask for an urgent blood test on the way out, that would be great. I'll write that down for you to give to reception.' I know DG has got a lot on his mind right now.

'OK, Doc, thanks.'

'Is that all clear then – are you OK with the plan, what will happen next?'

'Yes, I'll hear from the hospital within a week, otherwise I should let you know. And I'll do these urine and blood tests.'

'Is Mrs G at home at the moment?' I'd prefer him not to be on his own right now. Much better to be able to talk something like this through with someone close.

'Yes, she is. I'll chat with her when I get back.' Sometimes I give people the chance to practise what they'll say to their loved ones. It's a good way to check they've grasped what I've said, and stretches the value of our ten-minute meeting out into the real world. I judge, in a split second, that he would rather not do this. It's something about the 'I'll handle this' tone to his voice, and partly what I know of him already.

'OK, and you must keep in touch with us. Perhaps after the hospital has seen you, come and let us know what's happening, would you?'

I want to make it clear that we are not handing him over to the hospital for good. We are always here.

'Yes, OK. I'll come and see you in a couple of weeks; that'd be good.'

He gets up to leave. We shake hands. He gives me a tight-lipped smile, straight not curved, the sort that says he's trying to stay friendly and positive, but deep inside he's troubled. I return the smile, reflecting the same unspoken message.

(*thirteen minutes*)

Chapter 15

Master TB

*(**running thirty minutes late**)*

Doctor view

Appointment time: 9.50
Name: Master TB
Age: 2½ years old
Past medical history:
Nil of note
Medication:
None
Reminders:
None
Last consultation:
Ear infection three months ago,
requiring antibiotics.

Patient view
TB is a happy and thriving 2½-year-old boy. His mum works as a part-time accountant locally. TB is her first and only child so far. She has made an appointment for TB today because he has had quite a high temperature for the last two nights, along with a nasty cough which doesn't seem to be getting better. It's worse at night and that has been keeping her and her husband up, making both of them tired for work. Her husband suggested, as he left for work this morning, that she take TB to the doctor today.

She has tried giving him paracetamol, which brings his temperature down for an hour or two, but then it seems to return. She wants to check that this is nothing serious (particularly whether he needs antibiotics), and wants to know if there's anything she can do to help with TB's coughing in the night.

Next to each name on my list of appointments is also the patient's date of birth. I can see that TB is a young toddler. That raises my spirits a little. I enjoy seeing children – in medical terms they are far more than simply scaled-down grown-ups. They can make me laugh out loud, and their innocence means our interactions are untainted by the prejudices and complexities that adults often bring. It's often easier to empathise with children. They have a refreshing honesty that can make connecting and assessing them more straightforward. On the other hand, they can scream till your ears hurt, make you sick with worry, and turn dangerously unwell within minutes.

'Hello T. Come on in.' And to Mum: 'Hello, how are you?'

I know this little man, and his mum. They've been in before for minor stuff. That's another important feature of consulting with children – there are usually at least two 'patients'. She's a Sensible Mum – that's not an official diagnosis but it almost qualifies. I know it sounds judgemental, but I do have to consider that sort of thing when it comes to children. Of the two patients in the room, my overriding duty is to the child. A parent's ability to cope, and to make decisions in the best interest of their child, always has to be on my radar, albeit very faintly in nearly every case. These days all GPs have to attend formal child safeguarding training at least every three years.

'Hello, Doctor Easton. Thank you for seeing us so quickly. I made the appointment because T's had a temperature for the last two nights, and I'm struggling to get it down. Paracetamol works for a bit but then it comes back again. He's not "ill" ill. But he's got this awful cough and nothing seems to help it. Mr B and I just thought it was worth bringing him for you to check him over and make sure it's not anything to worry about, you know. Come up here, T, and sit on my lap.'

'Thank you. That's fine, yes, of course I'll check him over.' I turn to T.

'Why don't we have a look at these books I've got? This is a good one – it's got furry bits and shiny bits to feel. I think it's my favourite.'

I've now watched TB jump down from the waiting room seat, run along the corridor, smile, and follow my instructions. Now he's 'reading' a book, fully engaged with the fluffy bits, mumbling away to himself about monsters and showing his mum the pictures he likes best. I'm already relaxing – this is clearly not a sick child.

I spent six months of my GP training working as a paediatric senior house officer in a hospital. It was too short a time to learn all the skills of a specialist paediatrician, but long enough to get a handle on the main trick I needed to master as a generalist: how to spot a sick child. That may sound pretty basic, but it can be a huge challenge. I was on a steep learning curve. I found it emotionally tough and quite often I was scared out of my wits. There I was, in my mid-twenties, regularly resuscitating premature babies who were slowly turning blue because they weren't strong enough to take their own first breath. Terrified mothers ran into the emergency department to deliver their floppy mottled child into my arms, like a fragile express parcel. I watched over croupy, wheezy toddlers, fighting for each breath like an old smoker nearing the end. I even once injected adrenaline directly into a baby's heart to bring it back to life, like a paediatric version of the famous scene from *Pulp Fiction*. These were all shocking things, but they taught me about extreme illness and I think helped me to define the line between sick and well. In medical terms, that is the most important thing I learned.

I learned about my own limits too. We had a supportive team, and I just about coped. But there was one weekend on call when I crumpled. I started work on Friday morning and worked straight through until Monday afternoon, twenty-four hours a day. I had just a few hours' sleep in that time; even when my bleep didn't go off I was just waiting for it to shriek in my ear at any moment, like a furious sergeant on parade. We were busy, as always, but from memory nothing dreadful happened that weekend. But when I crawled past the finishing post on the Monday and got in my car to drive home, I dissolved into tears and couldn't stop for several hours. It was pure exhaustion – lack of sleep along with the relentless threat of a seriously ill child appearing at any moment. I admire paediatricians enormously – the ones I have met have been compassionate, skilful and wise, with the toughness you really need to be any use in a field like that. I learned a huge amount about children and myself in those six months. And I am delighted that junior doctors' hours are no longer quite so brutal and unsafe – although too often they are still dangerously long, recently becoming a source of bitter dispute between junior doctors and the British government, culminating in the first doctors' strike in the UK for forty years.

Fever is one of the most common reasons for a child to be taken to see a doctor and is the second most common reason for a child to be admitted to hospital. Most children we see with fever in general practice do not have a serious illness – less than 1 per cent according to one estimate. Most fevers are caused by a self-limiting virus and will get better on their own; but, of course, a few will be down to a serious bacterial cause such as meningitis or pneumonia. Despite advances in healthcare, including the huge success of childhood vaccination programmes, infections remain the leading cause of death in children under the age of five years. So I need to spot the one really sick child in every 125 slightly sick ones. That's hard to do because they turn up so infrequently, the signs of serious illness often aren't there early in the disease process when we first see the child, and the only diagnostic tools at our disposal are the old-fashioned history and examination.

One of the most valuable lessons I learned doing paediatrics was to listen to what the parents are saying. Really listen. Our consultants used to tell us: 'The parents know their child far better than you do – if they say something isn't right, take them seriously.' That was especially true when I was a junior doctor with little experience of looking after other people's children, and zero experience of raising my own. I always found it hard to advise parents about the more basic aspects of childcare like feeding, or what's normal poo and what isn't, or when crying becomes a worrying sign. I had been to the lectures (most of them anyway), but I had no real-life yardstick. In fact parents often used to ask me how old I was, which I resented because it reminded me of my inexperience. I was in my midtwenties but probably looked about fifteen, and once or twice even wore a friend's glasses in clinic to make myself look a bit older and stem the 'Blimey, you doctors are getting younger and younger!' comments. That's not so much of a problem now – with two teenage children of my own, plenty of grey hairs, and my own proper glasses.

As usual, I start with the history.

'So you said he's not "ill" ill – he's not drowsy or clingy. He seems to be playing as usual, does he?'

Perhaps the most useful information for me is this general assessment by a parent or carer who knows the child well. It's one thing when a child is a bit miserable; off their food perhaps. But when Mum or Dad says the child is not his or her normal self at all, not interested in anything, drowsy, or excessively clingy, that's different. Their eyes reveal the terrifying vulnerability you feel when someone you know and love is behaving like a complete stranger.

'Oh, yes, he's fine like that. And he's eating and drinking OK. In fact he's quite happy during the day. It's just the temperature in the night really, and the cough.'

Eating and drinking is a useful gauge of normality. I always particularly focus on drinking. Children can manage for quite a while without food – but when they are not drinking, or they are losing fluids through vomiting or diarrhoea, there's a real danger of dehydration. We need fluids and salts to survive. That's why, across the world, diarrhoeal disease is the second leading cause of death in children under five years old, and kills around 760,000 children every year. Most people who die from diarrhoea actually die from severe dehydration and fluid loss. Small children, like older adults, are at special risk of running dry.

'He's not had any vomiting or diarrhoea, and he's peeing OK, is he?' Passing urine is a good measure of hydration – the body is super-efficient at saving fluids if it needs to, so dehydrated infants don't pass so much urine, and their nappies are dry.

'No, he's not had any diarrhoea or vomiting – and he's weeing normally.'

'And has he had any other symptoms apart from the cough?' The commonest cause of a fever and cough in children is a viral upper respiratory tract infection, or a viral URTI as medics like to call it. The upper respiratory tract includes the throat, ears and nose as well as the upper airways of the lungs. So URTIs often come with a cough, sore throat, ear infections, and a runny nose. If several of those symptoms are identified, then the picture starts to look typically URTI-ish, and we have a focus for his fever. For now, though, I ask this as an open question so I don't lead T's mum towards any particular symptoms.

'Yes, he has had a snuffly nose, and he's been sneezing.' Sounds like a URTI.

'Tugging ears?'

'Sorry?'

'Has he been pulling at his ears at all?' I'm slightly in automatic mode now, using my well-worn phrases probably at too fast a pace.

'Oh, I see – no.'

'And has he been complaining of a sore throat?'

'No.'

'No rashes you've noticed?'

She looks at him a little anxiously, lifting his little top. 'No, nothing really . . .'

Most modern parents are really switched on to rashes, thanks to publicity campaigns about looking out for the rash of meningitis. They know about the importance of a non-blanching rash (one that doesn't disappear when you press on it, classically using a see-through tumbler: the 'tumbler test') as a potential sign of meningococcal septicaemia. It's a good thing to raise awareness, and non-blanching rashes do need to be taken very seriously. The trouble for me is that behind the simple public health message that 'a rash that doesn't fade when you press on it is likely to be meningitis' is a much more complex story. For a start, in an otherwise well child, most non-blanching rashes (as many as 90 per cent) will not be caused by meningococcal disease or other serious infections. A large proportion will be down to a simple virus that will get better on its own. Then there are several specific conditions that also cause purpuric rashes (the typical purple or red non-blanching rashes that sometimes also accompany meningitis).

For example, a condition called Henoch-Schönlein purpura typically causes a purpuric rash on the buttocks and limbs in children, sometimes with joint or abdominal pain. Then there are petechiae – small pinpoint non-blanching spots rather than the larger purpuric patches, which tend to be more than 2 mm across. There's a wide range of causes for petechiae, from infections to blood disorders or medications. Some are serious. But perhaps one of the commonest causes is extreme vomiting or bouts of coughing, where petechiae appear over the upper chest and neck due to the increased pressure in the thorax when you cough or vomit, causing leakage of blood from capillaries. Finally, meningitis doesn't always come with a rash at all, or it may develop only very late on in the illness. But, given that most deaths from meningitis occur within twenty-four hours, there is a very narrow window of opportunity for treating a child with the disease. So the bottom line is that parents *do* need to get urgent medical attention for a child with a non-blanching rash; and doctors always need to treat it very seriously.

'And waterworks OK? No tummy pain?'

'Yes, no problems there.'

Urine infections are at the front of my mind when dealing with children with fever. For babies they can cause serious illness without the specific urinary symptoms adults tend to get, like pain on passing urine, going more often, or abdominal or loin pains. For older children, there are often symptoms but they can present as vague tummy pain with fever. Once you have seen extremely sick children with urine infections it becomes almost second nature to at least enquire about urinary problems or tummy pains in a child with fever, and to think about checking a urine sample.

(*three minutes*)

'OK, shall we have a look at you then?' I say to TB, trying to sound friendly but not too creepy.

Examining children is a mystical art, like horse-whispering. I can't say I've mastered it yet. We have an advantage in general practice compared with our hospital colleagues – we often get to know a child well enough to build a trusting friendship. That can be like gold dust when you are trying to look in their ear or throat, or listen to their chest.

There are some tricks of the trade that I have learned over the years which make examining a child a little easier. For a start, talking directly to a small child as they come in can be too overwhelming for some. The 'jolly doctor' routine can backfire and many times I have ended up looking like a dismal clown at an over-ambitious children's party, with all the tiny guests in tears. It's often better to chat to the mum, even slightly ignoring the child to start with, and let them see that all is OK. I might notice a beady eye looking at me while I'm talking to the grown-up, and gradually, at their own pace, the child approaches this rather strange man who smells of disinfectant.

It's helpful to see the examination as a team enterprise, and get the mum or dad or carer to help me. Small children are often happier on Mum's lap, so we can do most things there rather than on the couch. I can show the parent or carer how to hold the little one for an ear examination – one hand firmly holding the head against her chest, the other pinning down any flailing arms. Some parents are brilliant at this and understand the need for firmness, even though it can feel a bit cruel at the time. If the child moves their head suddenly while my otoscope is jammed in their ear, I could do some real damage and our trusting relationship could shatter with a sudden painful jolt.

When I worked in Ear, Nose and Throat surgery in my training, the nurses were expert at taking on the role of firm child-holder as I prepared to remove all sorts of small objects which had been jammed up various toddlers' noses or ears. I remember a lot of Lego, and garden peas; just the right size to get lodged up your schnoz. The parents were often sent out of the treatment room if the child was too distressed. It seemed a bit harsh to me, but it was a relief. Upset parents just made the child more unhappy, whipping up anxiety levels in the room, and increasing the chance of having to go to theatre for a risky general anaesthetic. Sometimes the nurse would wrap the toddler tightly in a blanket like a giant sausage roll. It was tough love, and made my job a whole lot easier.

I start with something relatively unthreatening, and which the child is used to – for example, listening to their chest, or checking the temperature in their ear (these days ear thermometers are often familiar, homely gadgets). We listen for the bleep which says the thermometer is ready, and play a silly game guessing where the stethoscope should go.

'Does it go here, in your ear? Or on the end of your nose? No – of course not; on your tummy!'

Sometimes I get a giggle and we're friends. But like a mediocre stand-up comic, I do sometimes just get the stare which says: 'Get on with it, you idiot.' Sometimes my audience actually gets up and walks out. Occasionally, I listen to the mother's chest first, or look in her throat, or a sibling's throat, to show that it's all OK. That sometimes does the trick for the wary ones. My golden rule for young toddlers and babies, though, is to save the throat examination until last. Unsurprisingly, thrusting a lollipop stick down the back of their throat sets them off. Then it's really hard to listen to the chest or heart, and any trust flies out the window.

Temperature is up – 37.5°C. Slightly raised (37.2 would be normal for ear measurements). I check T's ears, with Mum expertly clamping him steady. All normal.

His chest is crystal clear, no crackles or wheezing; just smooth, clean breath sounds. While I'm there I time his breaths – his respiratory rate is an important measure of how much effort he's having to make to get the oxygen he needs. He's at twenty-five breaths per minute, which is fine. I'm also making a note of any in-drawing of the muscles between his ribs when he breathes – intercostal recession – another sign of laboured breathing.

I'm making a general assessment of T's colour (mottled skin, ashen colour or a blueness around the lips or hands and feet can spell serious illness) and any other signs of difficulty breathing, like grunting or flaring of the nostrils. His skin feels warm – not the peripheral coolness some seriously unwell children can have. I gently pinch the skin on the back of his hand to check skin turgor – if the skin is slow to spring back, it can be a sign of dehydration. Other signs of dehydration would be dry mucous membranes – eyes, mouth – or, in babies, a sunken fontanelle (a soft spot in the skull of babies which can act as a sort of barometer of internal pressure). If I was worried about meningitis I'd check specifically for neck stiffness and photophobia (sensitivity to bright lights), both signs that the meninges (the lining of the brain) are irritated. I have already seen T move his neck freely, and he's quite happy with the lights.

Still with my stethoscope on his chest, I listen to his tiny heart, naturally beating away faster than an adult's, and a little bit faster still because of his temperature and general discomfort. A fast heart rate can be a sign of physical distress – more than 140 beats per minute in his age group would raise alarm bells for me. He is beating away at 120, normal colour. Finally, I check his capillary refill time by pressing on the skin over his breastbone so it goes pale, and then timing how long it takes for the pink colour to return. It's a measure of the speed with which the capillaries refill after being emptied. A slow refill time can reflect problems with circulation, a pointer towards serious illness like dehydration or shock. Less than two seconds is ideal – his is very rapid, nearer to the one-second mark.

I've saved the worst for last. I ask Mum to hold him firmly, facing me, on her lap. And I start by asking him if he can open his mouth really wide for me. I show him what I mean.

'Aaaaagh!'

No joy. In fact his lips are tightening firmly. We try having a quick look in Mummy's throat:

'Mummy can say Aah,' and she demonstrates a real gift for it.

But T is still not impressed. I take a dreaded 'lollipop' stick from the packet and gently prod it towards his increasingly clam-like lips. He looks at me as if I am a very strange man invading his personal space, which of course I am. I continue. There's a tiny opening of the lips and I seize my chance, advancing the flat, rounded wood carefully but firmly towards the back of his mouth.

He gags. I see a flash of his tonsils. He starts crying.

I get an even better view now. Like the pain of ripping an old plaster off, it's horrible but the procedure is short-lived.

(*six minutes*)

256

'All normal, well done, T. You have been *such* a good patient. Would you like one of my special stickers for being brave? You can choose one . . .'

When I was doing paediatrics, I was taught to gather all this sort of information to make a proper assessment of a sick child. But a lot was left to my interpretation – I wasn't told exactly how fast a heart rate was too fast, or how high a temperature spelt danger, or how many seconds' capillary refill time was too slow. I suppose I relied on a rough sense of what was abnormal, and a nose for a sick child. Now, in the age of evidence-based medicine, there are guidelines from the National Institute for Health and Care Excellence in the UK (NICE) which spell it all out very clearly. The guidelines include a traffic light system for assessing risk of serious illness in children with fever. Green means low risk, amber is intermediate, and red is high (needing urgent face-to-face assessment by a specialist within two hours or sooner if clinically appropriate). The features of each category are clearly defined – symptoms including specific heart rates for different age ranges, respiratory signs and rates, activity levels, and other signs of specific diseases such as meningitis. It's a fantastic resource, particularly when a child is on the border between well and sick. It gives me confidence to refer a child to hospital, for example, when in years gone by I may have felt I was over-worrying. And on occasion it has allowed me to advise keeping the child at home, with careful back-up plans should they deteriorate.

On the other hand, there has been an interesting exchange about these traffic light guidelines in the *British Medical Journal* recently. An outspoken GP and writer in the journal, Des Spence, wrote a piece questioning the evidence behind the guidance, which now 'infects all areas of the NHS'. He has three main criticisms. The first is that the traffic light system is largely based on the opinion and interpretation of a small panel of experts. The second is that much of the research on which the guidance is based comes from hospital studies, where serious diseases are far more common than in the communities in which we GPs see children. Third, some work trying to validate the traffic light system found that it is not a very accurate predictor of illness.

The group that produced the NICE guidelines countered, saying that the panel was actually quite large and diverse, and that the guidelines were open to public consultation too. They also made the point that the studies on which the guidelines were based came from a range of settings across hospitals and in the community. And concerning the study that suggested the traffic light system wasn't a very accurate predictor, they claimed that this had not taken account of wider, more detailed guidelines.

What they both agreed on though was that, as Spence put it: 'Clinical assessment is in fact a rainbow coloured problem-solving affair based on experience, observation, continuity, and clinical intuition.' Interestingly, the guidelines agreed that when a child 'appears ill to a healthcare professional' this was to be considered a 'red' feature. I'd go along with that. For me, this is a neat summary of the pros and cons of clinical guidelines. On the face of it they are a great idea, and in some areas have smoothed out variations in quality of care across the country. They can be very useful in helping me make clinical decisions. But they have limitations – they are only as good as the evidence they are based on, and we clinicians need to back our own clinical judgement rather than turning into guideline slaves.

Judging by the official guideline traffic lights, and by my own internal version, TB is low risk. I'm almost certain he has an URTI.

'OK, thanks, T.'

I turn to his mother. 'So, his chest is crystal clear, nothing to worry about there. Ears and throat normal, slightly raised temperature at the moment. And I'm reassured by how well he is *generally* – eating, drinking, playing so nicely (until I shoved a stick in his mouth). I think with the cough and the snuffly nose and fever, this is most likely to be a viral infection, and I'm sure he'll fight it off himself without antibiotics and be fine. The key thing is to keep him nicely hydrated – plenty of fluids – and to give him some paracetamol or ibuprofen to make him feel a bit more comfortable. Don't worry too much about using those to bring the fever down – see them as making him feel more comfortable.'

'OK, that's great. So if I've given paracetamol and he still has a temperature a few hours later, what should I do?'

'Well, you could give him some ibuprofen in that case, if it's too soon to give him another dose of paracetamol. And, of course, it's important not to overheat him with too many clothes – you know, wrapping him up in lots of layers. What does he wear?'

'In the night?'

'Yes, and around the house?'

'Well, what he's wearing now. A vest, and top.'

'That's fine. Maybe he'd be OK in just a vest at night. That might help with the fever.'

'OK, we'll try that.'

'And the important thing is that I expect he will slowly get better over the next few days. If that's not happening, if at any time you feel he is getting more unwell, struggling with his breathing, or the fever goes on for say three more days, then come back to see us. Is that OK?'

'Yes, Doctor, thank you, that's great. You know I just thought it was worth checking. And what about the cough?'

'Yes, that's a nuisance. There's no magic cure for that, I'm afraid. Sometimes laying him so he is slightly head up can help. We don't generally recommend over-the-counter cough remedies for children under six any more – there's no convincing evidence that they work and they can cause side effects. So it's really paracetamol or ibuprofen, and drinking plenty of fluids, I'm afraid.'

'OK, thank you. Come on, T.'

'Thank you, T, you were very good. Bye bye.'

He beams at me and even waves. A fairly straightforward consultation. I carefully record all my examination findings. One of the benefits of the traffic light system is that recording of signs and symptoms in children has become much more rigorous – mine certainly has. When we used Lloyd George notes – little packets of loose-leaf paper – we would probably just have written 'URTI. Chest clear. Usual advice'. Not great for any other health professionals who might see him another time for the same problem, and deeply inadequate for the lawyers should anything go wrong. Always a consideration.

(*seven minutes*)

Chapter 16

Master RC

*(**running twenty-seven minutes late**)*

Doctor view

Appointment time: 10.00
Name: Master RC
Age: 5 months old
Past medical history:
    Born by caesarean section
    Premature birth 34 weeks
    Nil else of note
    All immunisations up to date
Medication:
    None
Reminders:
    None
Last consultation:
    A non-specific viral rash four weeks ago.
    Several visits for viral URTIs.

Patient view

RC is a 5-month-old boy who was born prematurely and who has been to the doctor's several times during the first few months of his life with various self-limiting colds and coughs. His mother lives on her own and has recently moved to the area, so doesn't have any family or many friends nearby.

RC had cold-like symptoms for about five days and has developed a nasty wheezy cough over the last two days. He is bottle fed but his mother is struggling to feed him at the moment – he just doesn't seem interested. His mother has tried her best to stick to the usual advice she gets when he has a cold, which is to give him paracetamol and make sure he drinks plenty of fluids. But she is really struggling to get him to feed and is now very worried about him.

The final whistle has been blown, and now we are in 'extra' time. At the end of each morning surgery I have three short 'extra' slots, which are kept free for emergency cases that need to be seen urgently, on that day. That doesn't always mean that they are what your typical doctor would classify as a medical emergency – patients often have very different ideas about what constitutes an emergency (for example, painful verrucas, long-standing muscle aches and pains, hair loss, sore throats that have just come on that morning, and so on). That's probably why, in our practice at least, the label for these five-minute slots has morphed from 'emergency' slots to 'extra' slots. But whatever they are called, they are short, each one should tackle just a single urgent issue, and there are only three of them. I feel as though I am now on the home stretch.

I reconsider my de-mob end-of-surgery mood as soon as I see little RC. My initial scan of him, sitting on his mother's lap in the waiting room, tells me he is not at all well. I am used to irritable, howling children, frustrated at the boring wait or hungry for their next feed. But RC has the irritability that often goes with illness – the desperate restlessness of not being able to catch a breath, of not feeling 100 per cent, of not being able to get comfortable. As I get closer, I can hear him wheezing, and notice a subtle but unmistakable blue tinge to his lips. He is 'head-bobbing' too; lifting and lowering his head in time with his breathing, a sign of the sheer effort he is putting in to sucking in enough oxygen and blowing out enough carbon dioxide. Normal quiet breathing relies on the diaphragm and the muscles between the ribs (the intercostals), but when breathing becomes problematic, people often start to call on muscular reinforcements – such as the accessory muscles of breathing, which are in the neck. RC's head bobs as he uses these so-called accessory muscles of respiration. (There's also the tripod or anchoring sign, where patients with breathing difficulties hold on to the edge of the bed, or children sit forward and clutch their feet to give them support for breathing.)

These signs are useful, and if I was using a diagnostic formula it would look something like: blueness + head-bobbing + wheeze = sick child with severe breathing difficulties. But there are other powerful clues that aren't so formulaic. The pleading look his mother gives me is one of them, and the way she looks at her son as if he is alien to her, not the boy she knows. I've also previously been used to her coming a bit late for her appointment, apologising with a playful twinkle in her eye, and chatting away about minor symptoms and last night's TV. Now she's on time and there's no small talk. In fact there's no talk at all as we turn back smartly to my room.

I've heard it said that doctors often make their diagnoses within the first thirty seconds of seeing a patient or hearing about their symptoms. That feels a bit rapid for complex or chronic problems, but it certainly doesn't seem way off the mark when it comes to emergencies. When the shit hits the fan, the usual order of medical things is turned on its head – a rapid examination, assessment and any urgent treatment come first, and the bulk of the history has to happen later, or in parallel. I do need to get the bare bones of the story from Mum, but I won't be dwelling on the nuances while RC is struggling away with his breathing. Children compensate for illness very efficiently (they can seem remarkably well when they aren't), so when they actually look seriously sick to a health professional, things are often grave and can deteriorate rapidly.

Because I can see he is slightly blue (called cyanosis) around his lips, and now at the tips of his fingers too, I know that his blood is depleted of oxygen, changing from the usual bright red to a much darker colour. It's usually a sign of a serious problem with the lungs (for example, asthma), the airways (for example, croup, choking or anaphylaxis) or the heart (in children, sometimes congenital heart defects). Given the wheeze and his head-bobbing struggle for breath I am thinking lungs or airways right now, rather than the heart or a more mundane trigger such as exposure to cold air or cold water (my son's lips used to turn blue after about fifteen minutes in a swimming pool).

Another big clue is the time of year. Doctors, like gardeners, must stay in tune with the seasons. In January in the northern hemisphere, when gardeners think about pruning pear and apple trees or repairing lawn edges, doctors are getting ready for norovirus (the 'winter vomiting' bug), influenza and bronchiolitis. Bronchiolitis is the most common lower respiratory tract infection in the first year of life: in the UK one in five infants is affected and 2–3 per cent are admitted to hospital. It's usually caused by a virus called respiratory syncytial virus (RSV) and while most cases are mild and clear up in a week or two without any specific treatment, some children develop severe breathing difficulties and need hospital care. In the US, RSV infection is responsible for the hospitalisation of an estimated 50,000–80,000 infants each year, the deaths of approximately 500 infants each year, and costs $365–$585 million per annum. The children most at risk of developing problems include those with heart or lung problems, the very young (under three months), or those who were born prematurely. In the northern hemisphere, bronchiolitis is most widespread during the winter (from November to March). So here is a child in the right age group, born prematurely, presenting during the bronchiolitis season, with classic respiratory symptoms which I have seen many times before. On this occasion, I am basing my initial diagnosis on the 'duck test': 'If it looks like a duck, swims like a duck, and quacks like a duck, then it probably is a duck'. Fancy medical articles about diagnostic approaches might call the duck test 'inductive reasoning': using observations as strong evidence to arrive at a likely (but not watertight) conclusion.

(*one minute*)

'Hello Mrs C. Tell me what's been going on with RC . . .'

'I don't know, Doctor. Look at him. He just isn't himself. He's not feeding at all – he's got this terrible cough. And this wheezing – I just haven't seen him like this before.'

'Yes, I can see he's not in a good way at the moment, is he? Has he ever had breathing problems, before? Asthma, croup, bronchiolitis, that sort of thing?'

This is a key question, and although I have his notes to hand, I want to make sure from Mum (often the most reliable source) that he hasn't had any of these problems, or any other chronic lung or heart problems, for example. I know croup and bronchiolitis are jargon words that lots of people won't have heard of, but a parent of a child who has had a serious bout of either will nearly always pick up on the words when I mention them.

'No, none of those. This is really unlike him actually.'

'Has he made any other unusual breathing noises – like grunting or "barking" perhaps?' Grunting can be a sign of serious breathing problems, and although I'm asking about the barking cough of croup (and imitating it, using my barking seal impression), actually parents nearly always mention that without any prompting because it is so unusual and striking.

'No, I wouldn't say barking or grunting really.'

'OK, and how did it all start?'

'He had a cold and, you know, snuffly nose, and then this cough started a few days ago.'

'What's the cough like?' We are slightly shouting to be heard above RC's noisy, wheezy breathing and crying. I am all the time watching RC like a hawk. He's certainly not in the mood for smiling. His breathing is definitely laboured, and he is not making eye contact with either me or his mother. It's as if he needs to concentrate fully on the job in hand – just breathing in and out.

'Well, it's a dry sort of cough, I suppose. We were all awake through last night because he was coughing so much. I just didn't know what to do. I gave him some paracetamol for his fever but it doesn't help really.'

'And how long has he had the fever?' My questions become more staccato, brusque even, when I sense an emergency.

'Oh – maybe two or three days?'

'And you mentioned his feeding – tell me about that. Remind me, are you bottle or breast feeding him?'

'Bottle feeding, because we had a lot of trouble with breast feeding at the start, if you remember. But he hasn't been feeding at all in the last few days.'

I need to get at the facts about his feeding, particularly how much, if any, fluid is getting into him. Poor feeding can often translate into 'not feeding at all' to a desperate mother, carrying with her the anxieties of the situation.

'When you say not feeding at all, has he managed any of his bottles?'

'Well, he has only taken a few mls of the last three feeds – I just can't get him to take any more. He's not interested at all at the moment.'

'And what about other fluids – water and so on?'

'Maybe the odd sip. But that's it really.'

'And has he been vomiting or had any diarrhoea?' I want to get a clearer handle on dehydration, and perhaps to rule out a different viral illness such as gastroenteritis.

'No, Doctor, no diarrhoea at all.'

'And are his nappies wet?'

'Not for the last – well, not since yesterday probably.'

'OK, thanks. And no rashes that you've noticed?' I'm saying this with as nonchalant a tone as I can muster.

'No, he doesn't have a rash – I looked. Or at least he didn't this morning.'

'OK, thanks. Well, can I take a proper look at him while he's on your lap there?'

(*two minutes*)

I move in to examine him, without stopping for pleasantries or asking consent from Mum or child. We all know there's no time for that now. But while I examine RC, I am talking calmly to him, saying 'well done', trying to sound chirpy. I may be feeling on edge inside, but everyone needs to hear some reassuring noises right now.

'All right, let's take this off, can we?' I'm keen to crack on with looking at and listening to his chest, gathering some firmer evidence to back up my instinctive sick child diagnosis. I want to gauge just how unwell he is.

While Mum is taking his vest off, I time his breathing rate. Sixty-eight breaths per minute. I know that's too fast, although I couldn't say exactly how much faster it is than it should be for his age. I'll check in a minute. I know it's fast in the same way that I know it's freezing when puddles ice over, without being able to quote the exact air temperature. He has some intercostal and subcostal recession too – the muscles between his little ribs (intercostal) and at the lower border of his ribcage (subcostal) are being drawn inwards every time he takes a breath in. To my eyes, those little rib-ripples tell me he is struggling. That's not normal for a child of his age and shows that he is having to create a larger-than-usual negative pressure within his chest in order to suck air into his lungs.

I warm my stethoscope between my hands, and place it gently on the boy's chest. With every out-breath there is a whistling wheeze, the air squeezing through the smallest-calibre airways (the bronchioles). Could be asthma, could be bronchiolitis. Even though he is crying, he is only crying on the out-breaths. So I can hear reasonably well during the in-breaths – there are crackling sounds all over, like a rustling paper bag. Typical of a lower respiratory tract infection, including bronchiolitis.

His tiny heart is tapping away urgently; I count twenty-seven beats in ten seconds on my watch. Twenty-seven times six makes 162 beats per minute. More than 160 beats per minute is faster than the normal range for his age. Another sign that he is in distress, his vital systems stretched to full capacity.

I take his temperature quickly, using an infrared tympanic thermometer in his ear, which shows 37.8°C (moderately raised). I don't read too much into the precise height of his temperature, though above 39°C at his age (three to six months) would be an 'intermediate risk' sign (38°C or higher in an infant less than three months old is a red-flag sign according to our current guidelines), and any fever that lasts five days or more definitely needs attention. He is crying, his eyes are moist, and there are no measurable signs of dehydration, but his lack of feeding and fluids over more than twelve hours, along with dry nappies, makes dehydration a significant risk.

I measure his oxygen saturation (the oxygen levels in his blood) using the finger clip monitor – 92 per cent. A healthy child without any breathing problems and breathing normal air should have an oxygen saturation reading of close to 100 per cent. Below 95 per cent is definitely a concern – and it doesn't surprise me, given his blue discoloration. When I check his capillary refill time – pressing over his tiny breastbone and seeing how long it takes for the colour to return – it's less than two seconds. So not too bad.

I am testing my theory of bronchiolitis against the evidence I have gathered. Could it be something else, like asthma, or pneumonia? Yes, it could. But with two or three days of a cold-like illness with snuffly nose and low-grade fever, developing into a persistent cough after about three days, the natural history of his illness is pointing towards bronchiolitis. The other tell-tale signs are the breathing difficulties he has now developed after three days, the wheeze and crackles in his chest, and the poor feeding (although that can be a general sign of breathing problems). He was born prematurely, which puts him at greater risk of developing problems, and it's the right time of year for this respiratory syncytial virus to strike. My money is on bronchiolitis, but I can't completely rule out asthma, or some form of pneumonia, or an element of either of them.

The main 'diagnosis' I need to make right now is whether RC is a 'sick child' or 'not a sick child', and whether he needs to go to hospital. The precise label takes a back seat. He is struggling to breathe, he is not getting enough oxygen, and he is in danger of dehydration. What his little body urgently needs is support with those basic physiological necessities – oxygen, perhaps some intravenous fluids, and the capacity for serious life support should things take a turn for the worse. Whatever the official diagnosis, the hospital is the right place for him to get that kind of treatment.

(four minutes)

268

My next decision is whether his mum can drive him to hospital, or whether he needs an ambulance. That's not a hard one.

'So, Mrs C, I've had a good look at R and, like you, I am worried that he is struggling with his breathing, and that he's not feeding properly – he could become seriously dehydrated if we're not careful. I think it's likely that he has a condition called bronchiolitis – a type of infection in the chest caused by a virus. Usually children get through it without any treatment, but occasionally it can cause real problems with breathing and feeding, and the best place to look after him in that case is in hospital. So I really think he needs to get to hospital as soon as possible, where the paediatricians can take a good look at him and give him the support he needs. I can organise an ambulance to take him from here. Is that OK?'

I'm actually just checking that she understands the plan, and making sure that she has been included in the decision as far as possible. I'm expecting her to agree with me. But this is not a moment for full-blown 'shared decision making' with the mother. Her child, in my professional opinion, needs to go to hospital urgently, and in an ambulance. If she disagreed with that plan, I'd have to insist.

'Right, OK. You think he needs an ambulance? Could I not just take him myself right now?'

'To be honest, I think he'd be safer in an ambulance, with any oxygen and so on right there. Can you see the blueness around his lips? That's a sign that he's low on oxygen, and we need to give him some here ideally. I'll get that started. But we can get an ambulance very quickly, no problem.'

'OK, Doctor. And how long do you think he will be there? Do you think he'll be OK?'

I can tell that this poor mum is now really concerned about her son – there's nothing like a doctor telling you there's something serious about a loved one to boost your worry levels. I know it would knock me sideways. I'm calm enough dealing with other people's children, but when it was mine, I fell to pieces. My daughter pierced her cheek on a thick hook-shaped necklace when she was a toddler. There was a bloody gaping hole in her face and she was making strange snoring noises through it. I threw her in the car and dashed to the local hospital. As soon as I handed her over to the lovely capable nurse, I dissolved into tears.

Sometimes, as someone who was brought up not to make a big scene in public, I cringe a bit when I have to make the biggest scene of all – telling a mother her child is dangerously unwell, summoning a huge wailing, flashing emergency ambulance to our surgery, and putting the hospital emergency department on standby. I admit there's a crazy, tiny part of me that would like to play it all down, keep the peace, and reassure her that everything will probably be fine. But of course that's not an option. Even if I am wrong about the diagnosis or have exaggerated the severity of this child's condition (which I have done on occasions), I would rather live with that embarrassment and the mother's irritation than the awful alternative. Actually, I don't think anyone has ever criticised me for calling 'action stations' when all turned out to be well. I imagine that perhaps once or twice the hospital doctors have tutted at me behind my back – the GP who panicked over nothing. Maybe that's just my paranoia, but I've been a hospital doctor too, and I've heard the sly comments about 'the GP', usually accompanied by some eye-rolling. This age-old petty professional rivalry between GPs and hospital doctors is improving now that more doctors have to spend time in primary care as students or during their later training, even if they want to be a super-specialist. Most of them quickly learn the challenges of general practice and come to respect the role of the generalist. But today's medical students still tell us that some of their consultants say things like 'You'd be wasted as a GP'. When you are a doctor in a hospital you make decisions with the support of a team of colleagues and specialists on hand, underpinned by almost instant blood tests, X-rays and scans, and with banks of hi-tech monitoring equipment and life-saving back-up just around the corner if anything should go wrong. I don't have that luxury. I relish the reliance on raw clinical skills and wrestling with uncertainty. To be fair, most doctors understand that, and most patients are very grateful that they have been taken seriously and that I have urged on the side of caution.

'Look, I know it must be worrying. I don't mean to scare you, but the best way to get R better quickly is in hospital, where they can do all the right tests and give him the treatment he needs. I can't say whether it'll be a few hours, or a few days – it just depends what they find when he gets there. But he'll be in the best possible place to get better.'

(*five minutes*)

I want to get the ambulance on the way and get some oxygen into R while we're waiting. Our receptionists are fantastic, especially in emergencies, and I go out to the front desk to ask one of them to call for a 'blue light' ambulance – in other words, an immediate top-priority call.

Once that's in hand, I ask our practice nurse for her help with delivering oxygen to the child via a mask. I catch her as she comes out for her next patient and explain the situation. We have oxygen in the surgery and regular training in how to use it – but children don't always appreciate having a mask put on their face, especially when they are struggling for breath. So this needs careful handling with the help of an expert – and emergencies are often best handled as a team. This child also needs constant monitoring until the ambulance comes, which should be within eight minutes according to our targets in London. I ask mother and child to go into the nurse's treatment room, and with the nurse's help we set up the oxygen at full flow and place the mask over R's face while he's sitting on Mum's lap. He is surprisingly amenable.

I'll pop in later, to check that he is OK, or when the ambulance arrives. But our practice nurse is highly experienced and will call me if the need should arise. In the meantime I start to jot down my notes from the consultation. I take even more care than usual on this one.

(*six minutes*)

First, the main presenting problem: 'Acute cough with wheeze'. Then I move on to the key features in the history: '5/12 [5 *months*] old, started three days ago with cold-like symptoms and developed into persistent cough with wheeze. Cough now disturbing sleep. Not feeding properly (bottle-fed) for last 12 hours or so – a few mls only each time. Mum reports "He just isn't himself at all." Fever 2–3 days, paracetamol not helping. Nappies dry last day or so. Born premature @34 weeks.' Then I record any relevant negatives in the history: 'No diarrhoea or vomiting, no choking. No hx [*history*] of asthma or croup or other lung/heart problems.' Now to the examination findings: 'O/E [*On examination*] Irritable, cyanosis round lips, also blue fingertips. Respiratory distress with use of accessory muscle, intercostal and subcostal recession. RR [*respiratory rate*] 68, HR 162. Widespread crackles and expiratory wheeze. Good air entry. Cap refill: <2 secs. Sats on air: 92 per cent. T 37.8. No rashes, photophobia or neck stiffness [*makes meningitis less likely*].'

I am writing this partly to gather my thoughts and build a coherent professional illness story for this little chap, but also for the benefit of fellow health professionals, including the paediatric team who I am about to call. Any doctor reading those notes or hearing them read out should hopefully feel that I have done a pretty thorough job in six minutes, and would understand the reasoning behind my diagnostic conclusion: 'Cough and wheeze with respiratory distress in five-month-old? Bronchiolitis.' Finally, my plan: 'Urgent admission to A&E. Blue light ambulance called at xx.xx hours. Paeds informed by phone. High-flow oxygen delivered by face mask in treatment room, under nurse observation until ambulance comes.'

I phone up the paediatrician on call in the hospital and explain that RC is on his way, trying to give a concise summary based on my notes. She's very helpful and says she'll be waiting for him in the emergency department.

(**ten minutes**)

I'm exhausted, hungry and still wired on adrenaline. I'm relying on a hollow energy that I've learned to use for emergencies when I'm dog-tired; like an engine running on fumes. I take a deep breath, rub my eyes, and lose myself for a second in my photos of the children. I double-click on the next patient.

Chapter 17

Miss GO

*(**running thirty-two minutes late**)*

Doctor view

Appointment time: 10.05
Name: Miss GO
Age: 25 years old
Past medical history:
    Urinary tract infections (UTIs)
    Tonsillitis
    Appendicectomy
Medication:
    Oral contraceptive pill
Reminders:
    First smear due
Last consultation:
    Urinary tract infection eighteen months
    ago

Patient view

Miss GO has noticed that it stings when she pees, and she's going to the toilet to pee more often than usual, too. She's had this for the last few days and it's been increasingly annoying at work. She has had three urinary tract infections over the last five years or so, and they all cleared up with antibiotics.

She has already tried the things she has read about in magazines, like drinking plenty of water and cranberry juice, but it hasn't helped. She called up earlier wanting an appointment for this morning, and was delighted (if a little surprised) when she was told there was one available. She is hoping and expecting to be prescribed antibiotics; she certainly doesn't want to be in this discomfort over the weekend, as she is going to her friend's wedding.

'I think I've got another urine infection,' she says with resignation.

I'm delighted. Not that she has a urine infection, of course – that can be utterly miserable – but that she has handed me the diagnosis on a plate. Some DIY diagnoses (the medical literature calls this 'self-labelling') are way off target. For example, one study found that patients often mislabel gout and chest infections as something else entirely. The trouble then is that I still have to make a diagnostic detour down the path they have suggested, only to discover after a few minutes that it's a dead end. Then I have to explain why I think we took a wrong turn, retrace our steps, and set off again down a different path. But some self-labelling is spot on. Tonsillitis is a good example, and patients seem to be particularly sharp when it comes to diagnosing their own urine infections. One study of women with recurrent urinary tract infections found that they correctly self-diagnosed 84 per cent of new infections (confirmed on laboratory tests). The key word here is 'recurrent' – patients' diagnostic accuracy seems to be linked to their own, or a friend's or relative's, previous experience of the same problem. I know Miss GO has had urinary tract infections before, so she is well qualified in DIY diagnosis here.

'Oh, bad luck. Does it feel the same as the ones you've had before?'

I want to hear her list of symptoms. Studies have shown that uncomplicated urine infections (cystitis) in women can be diagnosed very accurately on the basis of certain symptom combinations alone. The key ones are: passing urine more often ('urinary frequency'); pain or discomfort when passing urine ('dysuria'); a feeling that you really need to pass urine urgently ('urgency'); urine that is offensive smelling, cloudy or contains blood ('haematuria'); lower abdominal pain or pain over the bladder; and non-specific malaise such as aching all over, nausea, tiredness and cold sweats. The probability of cystitis in a woman with dysuria, urinary frequency or haematuria is about 50 per cent in primary care settings – the flip of a coin. When a woman has dysuria and urinary frequency without any vaginal discharge or irritation (which helps rule out problems with the vagina or cervix), the probability of her having a lower urinary tract infection (simple cystitis) goes up to more than 90 per cent.

'Yes, it's just the same as the last couple of times. It stings when I pee, and I'm going to the loo much more often as well. And I just have this general pain low down in my tummy, here.'

'Right. Yup. Sounds very typical, doesn't it? And no discharge down below?'

'No.'

'Any back pain, or pain high up in your sides?'

I have a textbook image of the urinary tract projected onto the back of my mind now. The urinary tract stretches from the kidneys at the top (one on either side), down through the urinary tubes (ureters) to the bladder and then to the outside world via the urethra, the urination pipe. Lower urinary tract infections, as the name suggests, affect the lower bits of the tract – the bladder and the urethra. It's also called cystitis. Simple lower urinary tract infections are benign and usually resolve within a few days. Sometimes they need antibiotics if the symptoms are severe or sound very typical, or there is evidence of infection on a urine test. But occasionally bacteria can travel upwards, to the upper urinary tract, leading to a serious infection of the kidneys called pyelonephritis. I have shadowy but powerful memories of women who have developed severe acute pyelonephritis; usually coming on rapidly with the typical symptoms of fever, rigors (extreme shivering or shaking), vomiting, and pain or tenderness in the loins (high up on the flanks, at the back, where the kidneys reside). Many needed urgent treatment in hospital.

'No back pain, no.'

'And you haven't vomited or had a fever?'

'No, I feel fine in myself.'

'OK, that's good. Right, well can I just check your temperature and feel your tummy quickly?' I rule out any high fever and make sure there's no loin tenderness. The guidelines suggest that someone with symptoms of a urine infection and either a temperature of 38°C or loin tenderness should be treated as if they have pyelonephritis.

'Right-o. That's all fine. So, what worked last time? You had some antibiotics, didn't you?'

'Yes, the antibiotics cleared it up pretty much straight away. I'm really hoping they'll do the same this time because I have my friend's wedding to go to at the weekend.'

'That sounds nice, where is it?'

'Somewhere in Gloucestershire. We're all staying in a hotel, and the wedding is in a beautiful old stately home – so it'll be very posh! I'm really looking forward to it.'

'Sounds lovely! Well, I think the antibiotics should do the trick pretty quickly. And you may be glad to hear that they're not the sort that react badly with alcohol either . . .'

'I was going to ask actually; that's a relief!'

In years gone by I would have asked her for a urine sample and tested it for infection using a 'dipstick' test. I know it sounds nerdy, but I used to enjoy that – the dipstick test involves a strip of card with several different-coloured square blobs along its length, each of which tests for something different. When you dip the card into the urine, the blobs change colour after a certain time if the test is positive. It is a miraculous mini-rainbow; complex chemistry on a stick.

One blob tests for white cells in the urine (one of the signs of infection), and another tests for nitrites in the urine (bacteria break down nitrates in the urine to nitrites, so if there are nitrites it's a robust sign that there is an infection – that blob turns from neutral to pink). But there are many other different-coloured blobs, for detecting other things like blood, protein levels, glucose and ketones, which can check kidney function and test for diabetes, for example. I love watching the colours change – an instant answer in pale pink. And for all the talk of new developments in rapid near-patient testing for all sorts of medical problems from cancer to infections, the simple urine dipstick is one of the few that we actually use every day in practice. But slightly disappointingly for me, we don't use it for straightforward cystitis any more because the evidence shows that it doesn't change our management if the patient's symptoms are very typical or severe. They need antibiotics come what may because, for them, studies show that antibiotics are likely to shorten the duration of symptoms by one to two days. Happily I do still get to dip urines when the symptoms aren't clearcut, or when people have only mild symptoms.

'So, it's called Trimethoprim, which you had last time. Just take one twice a day for three days. And drink plenty of fluids, OK? I'm thinking water, rather than alcohol!' I'm typing out the prescription as I speak. 'Ideally you shouldn't take these in the early stages of pregnancy – is there any chance of that?'

'No, no chance of that.'

The length of a course of antibiotics can be confusing for patients – and me. Some antibiotic courses are a week, some five days, some longer. But for simple lower urinary tract infections in women, a review of all the evidence has found that three days of treatment is more effective than single-dose treatment, and just as effective as five- to ten-day courses. All that happens if you extend the course is that you increase the risk of side effects. There have also been problems with the bugs that cause urine infections developing resistance to some of the first-line antibiotics. On the best choice of antibiotic, we have to follow local guidance that reflects patterns of resistance in our area.

'OK, yes, of course. And I'm taking cranberry juice and one of those sachets for the symptoms . . . shall I keep taking those?'

'Well, are they helping much?'

'Not really, to be honest.'

'I know it was recommended a while ago, but actually at the moment the consensus is that there is no good evidence to suggest using cranberry juice or cranberry products for urine infections is helpful, so I wouldn't bother. And the sachets that are meant to help neutralise the acidity of the urine don't have much good evidence to support them either. So if they're not helping, I'd stick to the antibiotics and plenty of water and fluids if I were you.'

'OK.'

'Your symptoms should be settling down over the next twenty-four hours or so. But obviously if they're not improving as expected, or if you get any fever or pains up in your loins – up here on your back where the kidneys are – then you need to see us or a doctor up in Gloucestershire straight away. OK?' Safety-net cast.

I hand her the prescription for the antibiotics and stand up – both signals that the consultation is now at an end. I am tired, and don't have the energy to explore any other queries she may have. This was a five-minute urgent appointment tagged onto the end of surgery so I feel within my rights to close this one down now.

'Yes, fine, thank you very much.'

'Enjoy the wedding!'

'Thanks, goodbye.'

(*five minutes*)

Chapter 18

Mr CP

(running thirty-two minutes late)

Doctor view

Appointment time: 10.10
Name: Mr CP
Age: 28 years old
   'Temporary resident'
Past medical history:
   No information
Medication:
   None
Reminders:
   None
Last consultation:
   None

Patient view
Mr CP is not registered at the practice but has asked to see the doctor today as a temporary resident. He says that he usually gets repeat prescriptions of oxycodone from his regular doctor but he has left that practice and is yet to register at a new one. He says he needs the drug for chronic abdominal pain.

He feels awful, sweaty and nauseous, and with some abdominal pain now too. He is desperate for the medication.

'Sorry to keep you waiting. I'm Dr Easton, come in.'

Mr CP smiles and takes his baseball cap off as we return together to my room.

'Have a seat. How can I help?'

'Yes, Doctor. I really need your help. I'm just down in London visiting some friends, and I've run out of my normal prescription for painkillers, and I really need some more, if you can help.'

I'm trying to place his accent – it's not a London one. There's a hint of Mancunian, I think.

'OK, and what is it you need more of?'

'Well, I normally get repeat prescriptions for oxycodone 10 mg tablets – they give me 112 of them. I usually get that every month, but I've left that surgery now anyway, and I really need some more today for the pain.'

I'm curious. He's being very specific about dosages and amounts. And oxycodone isn't exactly an everyday painkiller. It's a strong opioid, part of the same drug family as morphine and diamorphine (heroin). I have prescribed it occasionally in general practice – medically it can be extremely useful for chronic and severe pain, typically in palliative care but sometimes for non-malignant pain. Like morphine and heroin, as well as relieving pain it can cause euphoria; a type of 'high' caused by a surge of dopamine in the reward centres of the brain. It's this high that gives oxycodone a street value. Given repeatedly, opioids can lead to dependence. Opioids can also cause serious side effects, particularly when they are not used in the way they were intended to be used. Oxycodone modified-release tablets, for example, are designed to release the drug slowly and steadily over a twelve-hour period. But people who abuse the drug crush the tablet and swallow or snort it, or dilute it in water and inject it. This destroys the time-release mechanism so that the user gets the full effects of the narcotic in one hit, and hugely increases the risk of overdose and lethal side effects such as severe drowsiness and suppression of breathing.

'And what exactly do you take the oxycodone for – what sort of pain is it?'

I notice a damp film on his ghostly face – the pallor and sweating that can suggest opioid withdrawal. But they can also be signs of pain. Or anxiety. I am trying hard to keep an open mind – even if he is dependent on opioids, or abusing them, I have a duty to provide basic medical services for him. It may well have been us doctors who started him on it in the first place. Drug misuse is not only a criminal problem, it's also a medical one, and we're encouraged to think of drug addiction as an illness like any other.

'It's for chronic abdominal pain, doctor. They can't deal with it any other way. It's the only thing that gets to it. I've been taking it for a while now.'

'Right, OK. And can I ask about the abdominal pain? Do you know what's causing it, for example?'

'No one really knows, it's unexplained really. I've had all sorts of scans and that, and operations – look.'

He lifts up his shirt to reveal an old appendix scar and a midline laparotomy scar, running straight down the middle of his abdomen.

'What was that one for?'

'Exploratory really. Abdominal pain. The pain's really bad at the moment, doc. I do really need the oxycodone.'

'OK. Well, look. I do want to help you if I can, but I'm sure you'll understand this is quite a tricky one for me . . .'

When I'm feeling confused or grappling with a problem, I have often found that 'showing my thinking', a bit like showing your working in a maths exam, can be very effective. It allows the patient to see the balancing act going on in my mind, and implicitly invites them to engage with my dilemma, making it 'our dilemma'. The other overriding principle I am trying to stick to here is to avoid saying a flat 'No' right from the start. That can really wind people up – the medical equivalent of the blank-faced salesperson typing details into her search engine and coming up with 'Computer says no'. Equally I don't want to promise anything unrealistic at this stage, so I am trying to show that I want to help him if I can without committing myself to his specific request.

'. . . on the one hand, I do want to help you with your pain, and if you normally have oxycodone I can see that running out of it will cause you some real problems. But on the other hand, my problem is that I haven't met you before and, as you probably know, oxycodone is a very powerful painkiller with serious side effects and even the potential for addiction or abuse. So it's hard for me to prescribe it just like that, without talking to your own doctor, for example. It wouldn't be safe, wouldn't be responsible of me. Could you give me your doctor's details so I can talk to them on the phone perhaps?'

'No, I don't know the contact details. They've closed down actually. Can't you just give me the prescription – you can see I'm in pain. I've been taking them for years and it's never caused me any problems.'

He's talking louder, with a clipped impatient tone. He's staring straight at me, leaning across towards me. I'm uncomfortable. His story doesn't stack up. I've hit a nerve and we may be shaping up for nastiness. Remember the training on communicating with aggressive patients. Stay calm, professional. Try to see it from his perspective. Listen carefully, show I care, stay focused on a solution.

'Yes, I can see you are in pain, and I really do want to help you with that if I can. I'm afraid I can't give you that kind of prescription without any background – but maybe there's another way I could find out about your previous prescriptions for this: perhaps a pharmacy or something, another GP?'

I'm trying to stay positive, keeping a constructive channel of communication open between us. But I'm also setting clear limits, laying down the law. I can't just hand out prescriptions for that type of drug without confirming the medical details; I could do him – and me – serious harm.

'Look, I can't remember all that stuff and they won't be able to help anyway. This is ridiculous. I don't see why you can't just believe me. All I want is some FUCKING painkillers!'

On 'fucking', his fist slams on my desk.

'Are you saying you're not going to give me any? Is that what you're saying?'

His face is twisted. His eyes are bulging open, his mouth tight and his chin jutting. I'm much bigger than him, but I'm feeling threatened now. His shouting, his aggressive body language, and his unreasonable request for a powerful opioid make me worry that he will go to extremes to get what he wants. I had training in how to deal with aggressive patients when I was working in the emergency department. It often came in very handy in the alcohol-fumed, post-assault setting of A&E. But I've rarely had to use it in general practice. I remember learning how important it is not to escalate the aggression cycle by matching the patient's body language or voice. So I try to sound calm. But it's no good telling someone to stay calm – it just winds them up more. And it's confusing if you're talking calmly but your body language is telling a different story. So I keep my fists unclenched, avoid staring directly into his eyes, and don't challenge or humiliate him – that could be seen as aggressive.

I'm shifting into survival mode. I'm running on adrenaline now, my heart thumping, my vocal cords tighter, my voice a tone higher. Keep a safe distance, and make sure my exit route (and his) isn't blocked. If all else fails, I have a safety alarm which alerts everyone else in the practice that I need urgent assistance.

I learned the hard way about self-preservation. I was shadowing an ambulance crew when we were called to someone who had cut themselves. Rather than take the patient to the emergency department, I said I would stitch the wound in the back of the ambulance. While I was busy stitching, another person, shirtless and wielding a knife, jumped into the ambulance with me and started threatening me and my patient. I realised this was just phase two of a knife attack – looking back, the wound was suspiciously well defined, as if caused by a blade. Strangely, my reaction was anger because I was being distracted from my work, a kind of moral professional indignation. Fortunately, the ambulance crew opened the internal hatch from their driver's cab, leaned in to the back and dragged me to safety by my clothes. We locked ourselves in the cab and called the police, who seemed to arrive almost instantly. They didn't tell me off exactly, but they had very strong words with me about taking care of my own safety. Fortunately no one was badly injured, but it taught me a lesson.

'Look, I truly want to find a way to help you, but when you are shouting and thumping like that, it makes it really hard for me to help. Can't we work this out calmly – perhaps something else that could help with your pain, or maybe a local service that could help you?'

'I'm not going to a local fucking service. I know what helps, and that's fucking oxycodone. It's not difficult. You're a doctor, I'm a patient and I'm in fucking pain, right? Just give me what I need . . .'

He's now stood up, looming over me, pointing with his finger only an inch from my nose. I stay sitting down so I don't escalate things, but I'd feel safer if I was standing up – I could defend myself better and get out quicker. I'm turning from measured professional into self-defence expert.

I have tried my best to stay helpful within the constraints of my professional role. I understand that he is frustrated, but he is not prepared to consider anything other than his specific request. I can't just hand him what he wants without knowing much more. I now know that this is all about opioid addiction; he may even be dealing oxycodone illegally on the street. I can't be sure.

I'm angry that he's so aggressive. That has crossed a line. I am also aware that I am now what the guidance on communicating with aggressive people refers to as HALT – Hungry, Angry, Late and Tired; all reasons why I might be at risk of escalating this if I am not careful. I need to stay professional, and consider my safety (and that of others). I press the alarm.

'I've just pressed the practice alarm and all my colleagues will be in here any moment . . .'

'Fuck you. You pussy. I'm going to complain about you. Get you struck off. Fuck off!'

He takes a swipe at the air in front of me. I'm still trying to avoid confrontational eye contact, but now I get up from my chair and put my hands up to protect myself. I'm a good six inches taller than him, and considerably chunkier. I'm more an eating man than a fighting man, but I think he realises that his options are running out.

As I rise, he turns and marches out of the room, shouting 'Fuck' and 'Wanker' every few steps. He barges out, brushing past the first of my colleagues rushing in to my room.

I'm very glad to see them.

(*five minutes*)

Chapter 19

Finishing Off

The panic button summons pretty much everyone else working in the surgery, so it's a bit like a post-surgery party in my room for a while. Once it's clear that the panic is over and that I am OK, the main topic of conversation is how well the panic button worked. It's the first time we've had to use it in a couple of years. It's comforting to have everyone there, even briefly, but we all know this is out-of-the-ordinary professional socialising and, like schoolchildren enjoying an unscheduled distraction in a maths lesson, it can't last. We must get back to our hutches for some hard graft now.

I sit for a while on my own, head in hands. I am left shaken by the aggression. That's on top of the familiar feeling at the end of surgery – wrung-out and bone-tired. I notice the other usual post-surgery sensations too; a full bladder and a dry mouth. I haven't managed to have a pee, or a proper drink, for four hours.

Thinking back, I suppose the balance of cases this morning has been fairly typical for me. Some quickish follow-ups, a 'Did Not Attend', some regulars, prevention work, a few diagnostic conundrums, mental health issues, children, elderly with multiple problems, and a few lists. The last two emergencies were not everyday business though, thank goodness. The aggressive patient, in particular, stands out as a rarity in my genteel neck of the woods.

As usual there's been a fair dose of masterly inactivity (time is a great healer and diagnostician), empathetic witnessing, and listening. That can feel like you're not doing much – but the more time I spend in general practice, the more I am convinced that 'not doing much' is often the best thing to do. I think it's often more helpful than the modern trend towards over-testing, over-diagnosing and over-treating. I've made a handful of traditional diagnoses too – costochondritis, migraine, scabies, viral upper respiratory tract infection, and bronchiolitis come to mind. I'm not 100 per cent certain about all of them, but they are all labels with reasoning behind them. Time will tell if they are accurate. Then, as usual, I have set a few plans in train – further tests (for example, Mr EB with his fatigue and Mr WE with chest pain), referrals to specialist services (Mrs MR with falls and Mr EK with depression), and some starting, stopping or juggling of medications. As far as possible, given the time constraints, I've tried to do all this with my patients, as a partnership. The computer hasn't been too much of a bully today – in fact it has more often been an ally, warning me about prescribing risks, working out cardiovascular risk scores, as a prompt for discussion about test results. But I'm aware I haven't done nearly as much coding of diagnoses and template filling for points as it would have liked. I'm about half an hour late – not ideal, but given the cards I was dealt, I'm not going to beat myself up about that today.

My morning surgery represents just eighteen consultations out of more than a million every working day in GP surgeries across the UK. Each of my 43,000 GP colleagues will have had a slightly different flavour to their morning – over the years, the long-term GP partners might have collected more regular patients with chronic conditions, the stand-in locums might see more acute 'on-the-day' illnesses, GPs with a special interest might have had a more focused morning covering more of their expert area, like diabetes or minor surgery. GPs in different parts of the country can have very different patient populations, each of which has their own character. But whatever they have been doing, I imagine us sharing a collective sigh of relief across the nation at around 11.30 a.m.

I am sure another doctor sitting in on my surgery would have done some things differently; maybe point out a diagnostic possibility I hadn't considered at this stage, or a test they'd have done that I chose not to. A mistake perhaps. I am certain that another doctor would have used different turns of phrase and picked different consultation skills from their toolbox – many of which would probably have worked better for them. In a way that is the beauty of general practice, of medicine actually; you are always learning, and even with the pressure to stick to our evidence-based clinical guidelines, every consultation is different. General practice is much more than simple cookbook medicine – you have to be prepared to go off recipe, to season your dish according to each patient's taste.

I wonder how I've done this morning, and whether it's all been worthwhile. But there isn't time for the luxury of an internal daily audit, and in any case my memories of the first few patients are now growing foggy. I feel uneasy about not being able to call to mind all my actions over the morning – and, in fact, that uneasiness stretches back over weeks, months, even years. I make so many decisions each day and I must leave most of them where they were made, trusting that I did my best and laid robust plans. But I know that some of them will one day return from the past, ghostly reminders of an inexact science and my own human failings.

Sometimes it feels as though my patients and I have been on a white water ride, trying to stay afloat in the rapids of risk and uncertainty. It runs through every clinic, every day. I try to navigate by balancing probabilities, narrowing chances and sharing likelihoods. I've cast many safety-nets for patients, just in case. Guidelines and diagnostic rules can help me avoid major hazards. I even have my medical indemnity insurance as a lifebelt for when we're tossed overboard. Most of the time we make it through unscathed, but uncertainty and risk are constant companions.

One sturdy rock I can cling onto is my big red book. I've had to develop a sixth sense, an internal alarm which tells me when I need to check something, ask someone, or follow something up. Writing them down in the book takes some of the load off my mind. If there isn't time to make a note of them during surgery, I'll jot them down now. I am particularly concerned about the depressed man, Mr EK, and I must get on with that call to the mental health team. I take a minute to reflect on how I dealt with the child with breathing difficulties too (RC) – it all happened in such a rush. Of course I am worried about him, but now that he's in an ambulance and on his way to hospital I feel I can, and must, put him to the back of my mind. He is in someone else's care for now; in safe hands. I imagine

Mr DG going home to his wife and family, and what sort of a day they must be having. I wonder whether I pitched that conversation right. For me, our meeting was one consultation in a morning surgery – for him it could turn out to be ten minutes that changes the course of his life.

In my dreams, and in some of the tabloid press, once morning clinic is finished I'm free to have a leisurely lunch, play a round of golf or rush to the bank to count my money. But in reality this is when much of the nitty-gritty happens. It's now that I need to tackle all the tasks that have been generated from the morning: ordering investigations, checking and chasing results, making phone calls, dictating letters and navigating the Kafkaesque NHS system for referring patients to other services. Our long-suffering secretary tries her hardest to explain it to me each week: you can't use this form for that; he won't see anyone under eighteen any more; they only see people who meet these criteria; they won't fund those operations; we tried that once and the referral screeners sent it back. Our manic laughter verges on desperate sobbing.

As well as the stuff generated from this morning's surgery, there'll be the steady stream of longer-term tasks to get through. There'll be patient records to summarise (following patients who have moved from another practice), filling and signing health or life insurance forms, death certificates, cremation forms and mountains of repeat prescriptions. There are letters to write to schools certifying mitigating circumstances for exams, requests for certificates of fitness to take part in activities – for example, charity runs, marathons across deserts, or going on special commercial diets. Someone will have to work through the latest national or local health initiatives, making sure, for instance, that every person with a long-term illness or disability has a personalised care plan suited to their needs. We do regular audits of our practice performance too – for example, crunching patient data to see how we're doing with our blood pressures, or whether we're sticking to best practice in our prescribing. We all need to make sure we're ready for our upcoming Care Quality Commission (CQC) visit – CQC is the regulator for health and social care services (it's like an Ofsted visit for the surgery). One of us must make sure that we are on track to meet the performance targets we are set. There is always plenty to chip away at.

We train GPs in our practice, so I will often have to debrief our GP trainee once she has finished her morning surgery. She's a fully qualified doctor with at least three and a half years of hospital-based jobs under her belt, now spending the final year of GP training full-time with us in the surgery. At the start of their training year, trainees usually need thirty-minute appointments, but by the end they need to be ready to do the standard ten minutes. She talks me through each patient she has seen that morning, and a few she has spoken to on the telephone. She's several months into her training now – keen, up to date, extremely competent. Nothing like a looming professional exam to focus the mind. We whistle through her cases, I ask a few questions, make the odd suggestion. The learning is certainly a two-way process – it's always fascinating to hear how another doctor thinks. If we had more time, I'd love to debrief with other colleagues as well.

In the flu season we have a half-hour walk-in flu jab clinic to fit in; up to forty patients every day, divided out between all of us. I enjoy this – a practical, doctorly task with virtually no paperwork (a button on the computer automatically enters the details). It's simple, old-fashioned and uncomplicated; a healthy dose of medical science.

Lunch is usually portable and desk-based, competing with admin work. Years ago it was a more leisurely affair, perhaps in the company of others. But there seems to be no time or space for that any more. Communal coffee breaks, even seating areas, have been squeezed out by the urgent rush of modern general practice. Now we snatch debriefs standing at doors, and check how we all are as we wave hello and goodbye. Once or twice a week we have a practice meeting at midday to discuss clinical matters, practice business, and catch up with each other. It's a chance to share problems, and meet with other members of the primary care team like district nurses, palliative care nurses or health visitors. It seems like an oasis.

Now is also the moment when the duty doctor for the day distributes our home visits. Our threshold for visiting patients at home is now much higher than it used to be, but we do still do them. Where

I work, our average is about two or three a day – it'd be more in rural practices or practices with more patients on their list. They're usually reserved for the genuinely housebound who are unwell but not ill enough to call an ambulance or go to hospital. Honestly, I would love to do more home visits – I enjoy getting out of the practice and value the privilege of seeing patients in their own homes. When I do get the chance – plodding up the path with my doctor's bag, shifting the cat so there's space to sit on the sofa – it feels like an echo of a different age when there was time to really get to know your patients. I even remember having the odd cup of tea. But that era is gone. There just isn't the time or the manpower to do what my family doctor used to do when I was a child – pop in at the end of surgery when I had a bit of earache. We are just stretched too thinly. With travel time, I'd probably allow about half an hour for each visit – and that's in a suburban practice with a compact list area where distances are no more than a mile or two. In that time I could have seen three or four patients in the surgery. Home visits are also often done in dark and pokey rooms without all the equipment or the computer notes I'd like for an optimum consultation. So unless it's absolutely medically necessary, you're usually much better off coming to the surgery in any case.

I could really do with some rest time, a chance to recharge my batteries before the next phase of the day. But the patch between morning and afternoon surgeries is not a rest; it's really just a change of rhythm. As I work through my admin tasks or sit through our meetings, I am always aware of a looming deadline. I want to get as much as possible dealt with before the cycle begins again in a couple of hours with another eighteen patients for afternoon surgery. Otherwise patients' queries get delayed, urgent paperwork stacks up, and the day extends long into the evening. It's always a close-run thing.

The job has a perpetual element about it. The demand is relentless. I make my own punctuation points – start at 7 a.m., ten- or fifteen-minute chunks, two surgeries a day, admin, visits, home at about 6 p.m. Other doctors carry the baton overnight. But these are man-made divisions to make it all manageable. Births, deaths, illnesses, sore bits, worries, rashes, depression, pain: they are always there.

Sometimes I don't think I have made much of a dent on all that suffering. It's easy to feel like an admin clerk, wrapped up in red tape, having to prove yourself at every twist and turn, chasing pointless targets, and never enough time to give the sort of service I'd want for my loved ones. That is hugely frustrating. Along with the constant negativity about general practice in the media, rising complaints and demands from patients, increased workload and incessant political tinkering, it's sometimes hard to stay positive about general practice. I do understand why many GPs are fed up with what's happening, retiring early or going abroad. I've suffered from burnout myself in the past, and have had periods out of practice altogether.

But there's still something very special about the job – enough to keep us going back for more (and it's not the money, believe me). The huge privilege of being part of patients' lives at the really crucial moments. The trust that grows with getting to know someone properly. Sharing the authentic personal stuff – laughs, tears, fears, anger. The endless rich variety of people and problems. There's challenge too – enough complexity and serious medicine to keep the brain cells fully taxed. And every so often I believe I can make a difference. It's not always about dramatic diagnoses or emergency procedures. Much of it is simple and mundane – a sore toe, a rash, a worry, a blocked ear. Often the job is about absorbing anxiety, reassuring, caring, listening to stories of suffering, or just being there for someone going through a tough time. On a good day, it's an amazing job.

Follow-up

One morning surgery is just a snapshot in time. The value of general practice is that it takes a longer view. It's now three months on: here's what has happened to all the patients since I saw them that day.

Mr WE (chest pain)

He came back to see me a couple of weeks later, to discuss his ECG and blood tests. The ECG was normal. His blood tests showed only a slightly raised cholesterol; otherwise they were unremarkable. We talked in detail about how to reduce it through diet. His chest pains had disappeared. But this time he had a problem with his ear that was worrying him . . .

WE: initials inspired by Willem Einthoven (1860–1927), who invented the first practical electrocardiogram (ECG or EKG) in 1903 and received the Nobel Prize for it in 1924. This allowed, for the first time, the measurement of the heart's electrical activity for the purposes of medical diagnosis.

Mr NB (rectal bleeding)

I never heard from Mr NB again about any bleeding from the back passage, so I assume it settled down. Nor has he asked for any more haemorrhoid cream since that day. The bowel surgeons confirmed the diagnosis of piles. If I had been concerned, I'd have followed him up a few weeks later to check that it had settled.

NB: initials inspired by Napoleon Bonaparte (1769–1821), whose very painful thrombosed haemorrhoids (piles with blood clots inside) may have influenced his defeat at the Battle of Waterloo. Apparently they stopped him riding his horse and doing his usual mobile supervision of troop movements.

Ms AF (sore throat, fertility query)

She didn't come back about her throat, so I imagine it settled as expected. I don't know whether she cashed in her prescription or not. She did come back a couple of months later, with another sore throat, to see a different doctor this time. She was demanding a delayed prescription again. So I guess my discussion didn't make much difference, and I may have set an unhelpful precedent there for both my colleagues and me to live up to. Her fertility tests were all normal. At twenty-nine years old, with no relevant health problems, and having only tried for six months, I explained that there's no reason why she shouldn't be able to get pregnant. Nine out of ten couples in which the woman is under thirty-five will conceive naturally after one year of having regular unprotected sex. If she doesn't, I've asked her to come back then.

AF: initials inspired by Alexander Fleming (1881–1955), whose discovery of penicillin in 1928 has saved millions of lives and earned him a Nobel Prize in 1945, won jointly with Howard Florey and Ernst Chain. In his Nobel acceptance speech Fleming predicted the current global antimicrobial resistance crisis, caused by our misuse of antibiotics.

Mr NA (cardiovascular disease prevention, plantar fasciitis)

He had his twenty-four-hour blood pressure measurement, which showed his blood pressure was raised quite significantly. He decided to see if he could bring it down by losing some weight and watching what he eats and drinks; we're checking it again now (three months after the initial appointment). If it doesn't work, we've agreed that blood pressure medication will then be on the table for discussion.

But he's not really one for pills. He did get in touch a couple of weeks after the original appointment about his plantar fasciitis and asked to see a private specialist with a view to having an injection. I haven't heard any more about that. Don't know if it worked or not – but no news is usually good news.

NA: initials inspired by Nikolai Anichkov (1885–1964), who demonstrated the role of cholesterol in the development of atherosclerosis (furring of the arteries). His classic experiments in 1913 paved the way to our current understanding of the role of cholesterol in cardiovascular disease – and the development of statins.

Mr EK (depression, suicidal)

Straight after surgery I phone the on-call mental health team. It takes five minutes of listening to recorded classical music before I get through, and then another five minutes for a long and complex conversation about Mr EK. They say they will organise an urgent assessment for him at some point next week. I feel uncomfortable waiting that long; but they are the experts and I have given a full description of the issues. I have to contact him to tell him the plan; I'm relieved when he picks up the phone. He is happy with the plan. I tell him to see one of our doctors tomorrow, as a routine follow-up. I reiterate that he can always get help from mental health charities like The Samaritans at any time, or, *in extremis*, go to the hospital. A few weeks later, things have settled down and he is having regular therapy. But the underlying causes are still there; in particular, unemployment and isolation. We talk about those things over the next few visits and I signpost him to services that may help.

EK: Initials inspired by Emil Kraepelin (1856–1926), the German psychiatrist and founder of modern scientific psychiatry and psychopharmacology – the study of the effects of psychiatric drugs on the nervous system. He also inspired the psychiatrists who in 1980 radically revised the Diagnostic and Statistical Manual (DSM), the foundation of today's classification of mental illness.

Ms AW (sick note, back pain, abdominal pain)

The ultrasound of her abdomen was entirely normal. I am a bit deflated – I was expecting, perhaps hoping, that she would have gall-stones, which might explain her pains. But her symptoms settled completely over the next few weeks and have not resurfaced since. I checked all the usual blood tests, which were normal. I don't have any clear explanation for what happened. She came back again, twice, to discuss the pains and what might have caused them. Looking back, I think she was always worried about the possibility of bowel cancer; once I found that out and addressed it, I didn't see her again. I've told her that if it comes back again, which it may well do, then we may have to arrange an endoscopy to look directly into her oesophagus, stomach and upper intestines. If that gets us nowhere, she'll need a referral to the gastroenterology team for a thorough work-up.

AW: Initials inspired by Andy Warhol, the American artist, who suffered for years with gall-bladder problems. Apparently he was so afraid of hospitals, and so physically frail, that he and his physician kept putting off surgery until his symptoms became so acute that removing the gall-bladder was the only option. News reports from the time say that he had been making a good recovery from routine gall-bladder surgery but suddenly died in his sleep from an unexpected post-operative cardiac rhythm problem. He was fifty-eight.

Mrs JI (multiple problems)

Mrs JI had her ear wax removed, but the ear syringing triggered an outer ear infection which caused her some ear pain for a week or two. She wasn't pleased. I tried to find out about a new HRT medicine, and asked colleagues, but couldn't find anything relevant. The dermatologists didn't like the look of her mole and decided to remove it. Fortunately there were no malignant features under the microscope. She used her asthma inhalers as we discussed for a couple of weeks, then went back to her previous regime once things had settled down. Her son, Amin, went to see another doctor about his depression. That is ongoing. A few days after our consultation, she sent a complaint to our practice manager about how long she had to wait to see me. We discussed it at our practice meeting and I drafted a formal response, including an explanation and an apology, with the practice manager. Mrs JI still comes to see me.

JI: Initials inspired by Jean-Marc Gaspard Itard (1774–1838), an ear specialist in France in 1821, who was the first to describe irrigating the ear with a syringe to remove hard wax. He actually recommended using an enema syringe for the procedure; more specialised ear syringes were developed soon afterwards.

Ms JB (headache)

When she came back two weeks later, her headaches were still bad. She had tried the triptans twice, and they hadn't worked very well for her. So we changed the type of triptan she takes, and that seems to be working a bit better now. I didn't address her stress in the first consultation, but we have had time to look at that in more depth in subsequent appointments. It turned out that she was mildly depressed and tearful. I referred her to our local mental health counselling service (she is still waiting for an appointment for that) and she has also decided to leave her job and look for something else. That in itself has made her feel much happier, and her headaches have settled down a bit. In the meantime I have given her some self-help resources – an excellent book on mindfulness CBT (cognitive behavioural therapy) and a link to an online CBT course. I see her roughly every month at the moment.

JB: Initials inspired by Sir James Black (1924–2010), the Scottish pharmacologist who developed the beta-blocker propranolol, which is used, among other things, for the prevention of migraines. He was awarded the Nobel Prize for Medicine in 1988 for work leading to the development of propranolol and also cimetidine, a drug used to treat stomach ulcers. He was said to be a very private man, and was apparently horrified to hear he had won a Nobel Prize. He died in 2010, aged eighty-five.

Mr AB (did not attend)

He made another appointment a few weeks later. He didn't mention that he failed to turn up last time, and nor did the doctor. He doesn't normally miss his appointments. Fortunately his mole was benign and he was reassured.

AB: Initials inspired by Aneurin Bevan (1897–1960), coal miner's son, Welsh Labour Party politician and Minister for Health in post-war Britain. He spearheaded the birth of the National Health Service (NHS) in 1948, which was to provide medical care free at the point of need, funded by taxes. The current British government favours charging people for missed appointments to encourage them to take greater responsibility for the use of precious resources, although it recognises this would be hard to implement.

Mr GB (skin rash)

GB tried the permethrin cream according to the instructions. But two weeks later, he was still very itchy. His mother insisted on a referral to a private dermatologist, who confirmed the diagnosis and suggested an alternative anti-itch medication. The itching continued for another ten days or so until it gradually faded. In this case I doubt the specialist made much difference to the course of the disease – but it fulfilled a need for the patient and his mother, and that's OK by me if they pay for it themselves.

GB: Initials inspired by Giovanni Cosimo Bonomo (1663–96), who described and drew the scabies mite in 1687. Bonomo extracted skin samples from several itchy people and then observed them under a microscope to find 'a minute living creature … with six feet and a sharp head'. Physicians at the time weren't persuaded that such a tiny microscopic organism could cause such severe itching.

Mrs MR (falls)

I'm glad we got off on the right foot because I've seen a lot of Mrs MR and her daughter in the weeks since her first appointment. She has been to the falls clinic and they are doing wonderful work there with her. But she remains unsteady and has fallen a couple more times. I had a letter from the clinic saying they were worried she might be developing Parkinson's disease and would I consider referring her to our local neurologists? It was on my radar when she first came, but I didn't feel it was clear enough to refer her at that stage. Perhaps I missed a trick there. Or maybe we just had to let time take its course. Her walk has certainly become a little more shuffling since then. She's developed a more obvious tremor in her hands too. I look forward to seeing her, and she has settled in to her flat very well.

MR: Initials inspired by Moritz Heinrich von Romberg (1795–1873), the Jewish neurologist from Berlin who first described a test for sensory ataxia (unsteadiness caused by problems with sensory nerves) in the early nineteenth century (Romberg's Test). His family have a strong history in medical circles – his nephew was Eduard Henoch, who was known for describing Henoch-Schönlein purpura, a familiar rash in children.

Mr EB (tired all the time, TATT)

As is often the case, all his blood tests came back normal. Some people find that reassuring and that's the end of it. Others, perhaps with more persistent or marked symptoms, prefer to dig ever deeper in the hope of finding a single physical cause, a deficiency of this, or too much of that. But that's not always possible. Mr EB has subsequently had further tests for deficiencies, diseases and infections, and a chest X-ray into the bargain. I have not been able to satisfy him with my tentative explanations and theories. I sense a specialist referral coming on. The trouble is, for a general symptom like fatigue, which specialist should he see? We could easily end up on the secondary care roundabout, hopping from one hospital speciality to the next, each excluding any problems with their bit. I want to save him from that if I can. He may be the sort of patient we should discuss at a practice meeting – collective wisdom and fresh eyes often help.

EB: Initials inspired by Polish physician Edmund Biernacki (1866–1911), who discovered the erythrocyte sedimentation rate (ESR). The ESR is an easy, cheap, non-specific test to help diagnose conditions associated with acute and chronic (short- or long-duration) inflammation, including infections, cancers and autoimmune diseases. It's a measure of the rate at which red blood cells sediment in a blood sample in a period of one hour.

Mrs CH (thyroid monitoring)

Mrs CH returned in three months – her thyroid tests were all normal and she felt a lot better in herself too. She continues to be lovely.

CH: Initials inspired by Charles Harington (1897–1972), one time Professor of Chemical Pathology at University College London, best known for synthesising thyroxine and revolutionising the treatment of thyroid disorders. He was said to be shy and a little cold, but kind and generous too, especially to young researchers. He had a strong sense of duty and fierce intellectual integrity. He was elected Fellow of the Royal Society (FRS) in 1931 and knighted in 1948.

Mr DG (PSA: prostate test)

Unfortunately Mr DG's second PSA test was also high and a biopsy did show that he had prostate cancer, which had just broken through the outer capsule of the gland. Bone scans showed it hadn't spread to his bones though. He's opted for radiotherapy and hormone therapy and is doing OK on that so far. It's very hard to say precisely what the outlook is for him, but his urology team have told him that in men with his particular stage and type of cancer, between 70 and 80 per cent will survive for at least five years. I've seen him a couple of times since starting treatment for minor things, and just to touch base. He remains positive; we still manage to share awful jokes about golf, and his piloting exploits.

DG: Initials inspired by Donald Gleason (1920–2008), the US pathologist who devised a scoring system for the aggressiveness of prostate cancers in the 1960s – today, every man with prostate cancer will know their Gleason Score. It's based on the microscopic appearance of the prostate cancer – the higher the score, the worse the prognosis. It's been hugely influential in research and in clinical practice. His obituary says he spent his last twenty years sailing, baking bread and playing bridge. He died of heart failure in 2008.

Master TB (upper respiratory tract infection)

I haven't seen him since, and nor has anyone else at the surgery. I hope that means all is well.

TB: Initials inspired by Dr Theodor H. Benzinger (1905–99), a medical researcher in the US who developed the ear thermometer in 1964. He developed it while searching for a way to take a person's temperature and get a reading as close as possible to the hypothalamus, part of the brain that regulates core body temperature. Because the hypothalamus and the eardrum share blood vessels, Dr Benzinger decided to use the ear canal to take a reading. According to one obituary, Dr Benzinger once had electrodes implanted in his own hypothalamus so he could compare his brain temperature and the temperature of his eardrum.

Master RC (bronchiolitis)

I rang up Mrs C the next day to see how RC was. The paediatricians at the hospital agreed with my diagnosis of bronchiolitis (hurray). He had been kept in hospital overnight on oxygen, and given help with feeding. He seemed a little better the following morning. He continued to improve and was sent home after a couple of days. I've seen him a couple of times since then; Mum's not surprisingly a little jittery about any coughs or colds at the moment. But happily, he's fine.

RC: Initials inspired by Robert Chanok (1924–2010), the American virologist who in the 1950s identified and characterised the mystery virus that kills hundreds of thousands of babies every year – he called it RSV: respiratory syncytial virus.

Miss GO (urine infection)

Her urine symptoms settled with the antibiotics and she enjoyed her weekend wedding. But, like many women, she gets repeated bouts every now and then. At the moment she is managing just by treating them each time. We talk about what she can do to prevent them.

GO: Initials inspired by English physician George Oliver (1841–1915), working in London and Yorkshire, who in 1883 described tests for glucose and protein using paper or linen: an early precursor of the modern-day urine test strip.

Mr CP (demand for opiates)

The last I heard of him, he was stomping out of the surgery bawling obscenities at me, the staff, and any patients left in the waiting room. My fellow doctors were very supportive – there were several in my room within seconds of pressing the panic button. We had a quick debrief and decided to let the local health authority know about him. Sometimes they hear about patients who go from surgery to surgery requesting addictive drugs, some of whom may be aggressive, and they can circulate details to all local practices in case they should pop up elsewhere. What he really needs is regular contact and support with a local alcohol and drug service. We could have helped with that. I write up the encounter as a Significant Event for my appraisal and we discuss it as a practice, and what we can learn from it. We agree there wasn't much we could have done differently.

CP: Initials inspired by Candace B. Pert (1946–2013), the American neuroscientist who in 1973 discovered the opiate receptor – which we now know is the cellular docking site in the brain for the body's natural painkillers, opiates like endorphins. She is quoted as saying: 'God presumably did not put an opiate receptor in our brains so that we could eventually discover how to get high with opium.' She died in 2013.

References and Further Reading

Preface

Davis, K., K. Stremikis, C. Schoen and D. Squires (2004), *Mirror, Mirror on the Wall, 2014 Update: How the US Health Care System Compares Internationally.* The Commonwealth Fund, June 2014.

Chapter 1 (Chest pain)

Beckman, H. B. and R. M. Frankel (1984), 'The Effect of Physician Behavior on the Collection of Data', *Annals of Internal Medicine*, 101(5): 692–6.

Danczak, A. (2015), 'British GPs Keep Going for Longer: Is the 12-second Interruption History?', *British Medical Journal*, 351: h6136.

Marvel, M. K., R. M. Epstein, K. Flowers and H. B. Beckman (1999), 'Soliciting the Patient's Agenda: Have We Improved?', *Journal of the American Medical Association*, 281(3): 283–7.

National Institute for Health and Care Excellence (NICE) (2015), 'Clinical Knowledge Summaries: Chest Pain – Diagnosis', last revised April 2015; http://cks.nice.org.uk/chest-pain#!diagnosis

Neighbour, R. (2004), *The Inner Consultation: How to Develop an Effective and Intuitive Consulting Style*, 2nd edn., Radcliffe Medical Press.

Nilsson, S., M. Scheike, D. Engblom, L.-G. Karlsson, S. Mölstad, I. Akerlind, K. Ortoft and E. Nylander (2003), 'Chest Pain and Ischaemic Heart Disease in Primary Care', *British Journal of General Practice*, 53(490): 378–82.

Pendleton, D., T. Schofield, P. Tate and P. Havelock (2003), *The Consultation: An Approach to Learning and Teaching*, Oxford: Oxford University Press.

Chapter 2 (Rectal bleeding)

Allemani, C., H. K. Weir, H. Carreira, R. Harewood, D. Spika, X. S. Wang, F. Bannon, J. V. Ahn, C. J. Johnson, A. Bonaventure and R. Marcos-Gragera (2015), 'Global Surveillance of Cancer Survival 1995–2009: Analysis of Individual Data for 25,676,887 Patients from 279 Population-based Registries in 67 Countries (CONCORD-2)', *The Lancet*, 385(9972): 977–1010.

Coldicott, Y., C. Pope and C. Roberts (2003), 'The Ethics of Intimate

Examinations: Teaching Tomorrow's Doctors', *British Medical Journal*, 326(7380): 97–101.

Granados, A., E. Mayer, C. Norton, D. Ellis, M. Mobasheri, N. Low-Beer, J. Higham, R. Kneebone and F. Bello (2014), 'Haptics Modelling for Digital Rectal Examinations', in *Biomedical Simulation*, ed. Fernando Bello and Stephane Cotin, Springer International Publishing, pp. 40–9.

National Institute for Health and Care Excellence (NICE) (2015), 'Referral Guidelines for Suspected Cancer', June 2015.

National Institute for Health and Care Excellence (NICE) (2015), 'Referral Guidelines for Suspected Cancer: Appendix F – Evidence Review', updated June, pp. 504–616.

Chapter 3 (Sore throat, fertility query)

Ashworth, M., P. White, H. Jongsma, P. Schofield and D. Armstrong (2015), 'Antibiotic Prescribing and Patient Satisfaction in Primary Care in England: Cross-sectional Analysis of National Patient Survey Data and Prescribing Data', *British Journal of General Practice*, bjgpjan-2016.

Berne, E. (1968). *Games People Play: The Psychology of Human Relationships*, Vol. 2791, Harmondsworth, UK: Penguin.

Bourne, T., L. Wynants, M. Peters, C. Van Audenhove, D. Timmerman, B. Van Calsterand, M. Jalmbrant (2015), 'The Impact of Complaints Procedures on the Welfare, Health and Clinical Practise of 7926 Doctors in the UK: A Cross-sectional Survey', *British Medical Journal Open*, 5(1): e006687.

Greenhalgh, T., C. Helman and A. M. M. Chowdhury (1998), 'Health Beliefs and Folk Models of Diabetes in British Bangladeshis: A Qualitative Study', *British Medical Journal*, 316(7136): 978–83.

Heneghan, C., P. Glasziou, M. Thompson, P. Rose, J. Balla, D. Lasserson, C. Scott and R. Perera (2009), 'Diagnostic Strategies Used in Primary Care', *British Medical Journal*, 338: 1003–6.

Little, P., F. D. Hobbs, M. Moore, et al. (2013), 'Clinical Score and Rapid Antigen Detection Test to Guide Antibiotic Use for Sore Throats: Randomised Controlled Trial of PRISM (Primary Care Streptococcal Management)', *British Medical Journal* (10 October), 347: f5806.doi: 10.1136/bmj.f5806.

Little, P., M. Moore, J. Kelly, I. Williamson, G. Leydon, L. McDermott, M. Mullee and B. Stuart (2014), 'Delayed Antibiotic Prescribing Strategies for Respiratory Tract Infections in Primary Care: Pragmatic, Factorial, Randomised Controlled Trial', *British Medical Journal*, 348: g1606.

National Institute for Health and Care Excellence (NICE) (2015), 'Clinical Knowledge Summaries: Sore Throat – Acute Management', last revised July 2015; http://cks.nice.org.uk/sore-throat-acute#!scenario

Zola, I. K. (1973), 'Pathways to the Doctor: From Person to Patient', *Social Science & Medicine*, 7(9): 677–89.

Chapter 4 (Cardiovascular disease prevention)

Finegold, J. A., C. H. Manisty, B. Goldacre, et al. (2014), 'What Proportion of Symptomatic Side Effects in Patients Taking Statins are Genuinely Caused by the Drug? Systematic Review of Randomised Placebo-controlled Trials to Aid Individual Patient Choice', *European Journal of Preventive Cardiology*, 21(4) (2014): 464–74, published online 12 March.

Marshall, M. and J. Bibby (2011), 'Supporting Patients to Make the Best Decisions', *British Medical Journal*, 342: d2117.

National Institute for Health and Care Excellence (NICE) 2014, 'Cardiovascular Disease: Risk Assessment and Reduction, Including Lipid Modification,' NICE guideline [CG181], July 2014.

National Institute for Health and Care Excellence (2014), 'Lipid Modification: Cardiovascular Risk Assessment and the Modification of Blood Lipids for the Primary and Secondary Prevention of Cardiovascular Disease', NICE guideline draft for consultation, 12 February; http://guidance.nice.org.uk/CG/WaveR/123

NICE.org.uk (2014), NICE statin letter: 'Concerns about the Latest NICE Draft Guidance on Statins', 10 June; https://www.nice.org.uk/Media/Default/News/NICE-statin-letter.pdf

Prochaska, J. O. D. and C. Carlo (1983), 'Stages and Processes of Self-change of Smoking: Toward an Integrative Model of Change', *Journal of Consulting and Clinical Psychology*, 51(3) (June): 390–5.

Storr, E. (2011), 'Motivational Interviewing: A Positive Approach', *InnovAiT* (the RCGP Journal for Associates in Training), 4(9): 533–8.

Chapter 5 (Depression)

Anderson, I. M., I. N. Ferrier, R. C. Baldwin, et al. (2008), 'Evidence-based Guidelines for Treating Depressive Disorders with Antidepressants: A Revision of the 2000 British Association for Psychopharmacology Guidelines', *Journal of Psychopharmacology*, 22(4): 343–96.

National Institute for Health and Care Excellence (NICE) (2015), 'Clinical Knowledge Summaries: Depression', last revised October 2015; http://cks.nice.org.uk/depression#!topicsummary

Taylor, D., C. Paton and S. Kapur (2012), *The Maudsley Prescribing Guidelines*, 11th edn, London: Informa Healthcare.

Chapter 7 (Multiple problems)

National Institute for Health and Care Excellence (NICE) (2011), 'Clinical Knowledge Summaries: Melanoma and Pigmented Lesions – Assessment of the Lesion', Last revised March 2011; http://cks.nice.org.uk/melanoma-and-pigmented-lesions#!diagnosissub

Salisbury, C., S. Procter, K. Stewart, L. Bowen, S. Purdy, M. Ridd, J. Valderas, T. Blakeman and D. Reeves (2013), 'The Content of General Practice Consultations: Cross-sectional Study Based on VideoRecordings', *British Journal of General Practice*, 63(616): e751–9.

Verma, A., H. Bhatt, P. Booton, R. Kneebone, et al. (2011), 'The Ventriloscope (R) as an Innovative Tool for Assessing Clinical Examination Skills: Appraisal of a Novel Method of Simulating Auscultatory Findings', *Medical Teacher*, 33: E388–96.

Chapter 8 (Headache)

Alper, B. S., J. A. Hand, S. G. Elliott, et al. (2004), 'How Much Effort is Needed to Keep Up with the Literature Relevant for Primary Care?' *Journal of the Medical Library Association*, 92(4): 429–37.

Helman, C. G. (2007), *Culture, Health and Illness,* CRC Press.

Hojat, M., D. Z. Louis, F. W. Markham, R. Wender, C. Rabinowitz and J. S. Gonnella (2011), 'Physicians' Empathy and Clinical Outcomes for Diabetic Patients', *Academic Medicine*, 86(3): 359–64.

Hojat, M., S. Mangione, T. J. Nasca, S. Rattner, J. B. Erdmann, J. S. Gonnella and M. Magee (2004), 'An Empirical Study of Decline in Empathy in Medical School', *Medical Education*, 38(9): 934–41.

Launer, J. (2002), *Narrative-based Primary Care: A Practical Guide*, Oxford, Radcliffe Publishing.

National Institute for Health and Care Excellence (NICE) (2015), 'Clinical Knowledge Summaries: Migraine in Adults', last revised October 2015; http://cks.nice.org.uk/migraine#!scenario

Neumann, M., F. Edelhäuser, D. Tauschel, M. R. Fischer, M. Wirtz, C. Woopen, A. Haramati and C. Scheffer (2011), 'Empathy Decline and its Reasons: A Systematic Review of Studies with Medical Students and Residents', *Academic Medicine*, 86(8): 996–1009.

Roff, S. (2015), 'Reconsidering the "Decline" of Medical Student Empathy as Reported in Studies using the Jefferson Scale of Physician Empathy: Student Version (JSPE-S)', *Medical Teacher* 37(8): 783–6.

Chapter 9 (Did not attend)

Easton, G. and R. Baker (2015), 'Seven Days a Week, 8 AM to 8 PM: Improving Access to National Health Service Primary Care', *Journal of Ambulatory Care Management*, 38: 16–24.

Neal, R. D., M. Hussain-Gambles, V. L. Allgar, D. A. Lawlor and O. Dempsey (2005), 'Reasons for and Consequences of Missed Appointments in General Practice in the UK: Questionnaire Survey and Prospective Review of Medical Records', *BMC Family Practice*, 6(1): 47.

Royal College of General Practitioners (2013), 'The 2022 GP: Compendium of Evidence', London; http://www.rcgp.org.uk/policy/rcgp-policy-areas/-/media/Files/Policy/A-Z-policy/The-2022-GP-Compendium-of-Evidence.ashx

Chapter 10 (Skin rash)

Currier, R. W., S. F. Walton and B. J. Currie (2011), 'Scabies in Animals and Humans: History, Evolutionary Perspectives, and Modern Clinical Management', *Annals of the New York Academy of Sciences*, 1230(1): E50–60.

Friedman, R. (1941), *Scabies: Civil and Military*, New York: Froben Press.

Karthikeyan, K. (2005), 'Treatment of Scabies: Newer Perspectives', *Postgraduate Medical Journal*, 81(951): 7–11.

O'Donnell, C. A. (2000), 'Variation in GP Referral Rates: What Can We Learn from the Literature?' *Family Practice*, 17(6): 462–71.

Sherif, J. et al. (2015), *Using Arts-based Observational Skills Training, Modelling and Simulation to Teach Clinical Observation in Dermatology*, Association for Medical Education in Europe (AMEE) 2015 conference abstract book; http://www.amee.org/getattachment/amee-news/AMEE-2015-Abstract-Book/Final-Abstract-Book-as-at-3-SEptember-2015.pdf

Chapter 11 (Falls)

Age UK: http://www.ageuk.org.uk/professional-resources-home/services-and-practice/health-and-wellbeing/falls-prevention-resources/ (accessed 13 February 2016).

Avery, A. J., S. Rodgers, B. D. Franklin, R. A. Elliott, R. Howard, S. P. Slight, G. Swanwick, R. Knox, G. Gookey, N. Barber, et al. (2014), 'Research into Practice: Safe Prescribing', *British Journal of General Practice*, 64(622): 259–61.

Darowski, A., Dwight, J., Reynolds (2011), *Medicines and Falls in Hospital: Guidance Sheet*, London, Royal College of Physicians.

Gnjidic, D., D. G. L. Couteur and S. N. Hilmer (2014), 'Discontinuing Drug Treatments', *British Medical Journal*, 349: g7013.

National Institute for Health and Care Excellence (NICE) (2013), 'Falls in Older People: Assessing Risk and Prevention', NICE guidelines [CG161], June 2013.

Romberg, M. H. (1853), *A Manual of the Nervous Diseases of Man*, Vol. 2 (E. H. Sievekingtrans), London, Sydenham Society, pp. 395–401.

Chapter 12 (Tired all the time TATT)

Bellis, M. A., K. Hughes, P. A. Cook and M. Morleo (2009), 'Off Measure: How We Underestimate the Amount We Drink', Liverpool: Centre for Public Health, Liverpool John Moores University.

Groves, J. E. (1978), 'Taking Care of the Hateful Patient', *New England Journal of Medicine*, 298(16): 883–7.

Hamilton, W., J. Watson and A. Round (2010), 'Rational Testing: Investigating Fatigue in Primary Care', *British Medical Journal*, 341(7771): 502–4.

Heneghan, C., P. Glasziou, M. Thompson, P. Rose, J. Balla, D. Lasserson, C. Scott and R. Perera (2009), 'Diagnostic Strategies used in Primary Care', *British Medical Journal*, 338: 1003–6.

Mathers, N., Jones, N. & Hannay, D., (1995), 'Heartsick Patiients'. A study of their general practitioners, B,J Gen Pract, 45(395), 293–6.

Moncrieff, G. and J. Fletcher (2007), '10-minute Consultation: Tiredness', *British Medical Journal*, 334(7605): 1221.

National Institute for Health and Care Excellence (NICE) (2015), 'Clinical Knowledge Summaries: Tiredness/Fatigue in Adults', last revised February 2015; http://cks.nice.org.uk/tirednessfatigue-in-adults#!topicsummary

O'Dowd, T. (1988), 'Five Years of Heartsink Patients in General Practice', *British Medical Journal*, 297(6647): 528–30.

Chapter 13 (Thyroid)

DOI: http://dx.doi.org/10.1787/health_glance_eur-2014-26-en

Easten, G. (2011), 'Fifteen Minutes With the Patient, Please', *BMJ Careers*, 128–9.

National Institute for Health and Care Excellence (NICE) (2011), 'Clinical Knowledge Summaries: Hypothyroidism Management – Scenario: Overt Hypothyrodism', last revised February 2011; http://cks.nice.org.uk/hypothyroidism#!scenario:2

OECD/European Union (2014), 'Consultations with Doctors', in *Health at a Glance: Europe 2014*, Paris: OECD Publishing.

Okosieme, O., J. Gilbert, P. Abraham, K. Boelaert, C. Dayan, M. Gurnell and G. Williams (2015), 'Management of Primary Hypothyroidism: Statement by the British Thyroid Association Executive Committee', *Clinical Endocrinology*; http://www.btf-thyroid.org/images/documents/BTA_Hypothyroidism_Statement.pdf

Royal College of General Practitioners ((2013), 'The 2022 GP: Compendium of Evidence', London; http://www.rcgp.org.uk/policy/rcgp-policy-areas/~/media/Files/Policy/A-Z-policy/The-2022-GP-Compendium-of-Evidence.ashx

Wiersinga, W. M., L. Duntas, V. Fadeyev, B. Nygaard and M. P. Vanderpump (2012), 'ETA Guidelines: The Use of L-T4+ L-T3 in the Treatment of Hypothyroidism', *European Thyroid Journal*, 1(2): 55–71.

Chapter 14 (Prostate cancer test)

Baile, W. F., R. Buckman, R. Lenzie, G. Glober, E. A. Beale and P. Kudelka (2000), 'SPIKES – a six-step protocol for delivering bad news: application to the patient with cancer', *The Oncologist, 5* (4), 302 –311.

Public Health England (2015), 'Prostate Cancer Risk Management Programme: Overview'; https://www.gov.uk/guidance/prostate-cancer-risk-management-programme-overview

Chapter 15 (Upper respiratory tract infection)

Richardson, M. and M. Lakhanpaul (2013), 'Assessment and Initial Management of Feverish Illness in Children Younger than 5 Years: Summary of Updated NICE Guidance', *British Medical Journal*, 346(7604): 1163–4.

Spence, D. (2014), 'Bad Medicine: NICE's Traffic Light System for Febrile Children', *British Medical Journal*, 348: g2056.

Chapter 16 (Bronchiolitis)

Fleming, S., P. Gill, C. Jones, J. A. Taylor, A. Van den Bruel, C. Heneghan and M. Thompson (2015), 'Validity and Reliability of Measurement of Capillary Refill Time in Children: A Systematic Review', *Archives of Disease in Childhood*, 100(3): 239–49.

Ricci, V., V. D. Nunes, M. S. Murphy and S. Cunningham (2015), 'Bronchiolitis in Children: Summary of NICE Guidance', *British Medical Journal*, 350: h2305.

Chapter 17 (Urine infection)

Gupta, K., T. M. Hooton, P. L. Roberts and W. E. Stamm (2001), 'Patient-initiated Treatment of Uncomplicated Recurrent Urinary Tract Infections in Young Women', *Annals of Internal Medicine*, 135(1): 9–16.

National Institute for Health and Care Excellence (NICE) (2015), 'Clinical Knowledge Summaries: Urinary Tract Infection (Lower) – Women', last revised July 2015; http://cks.nice.org.uk/urinary-tract-infection-lower-women

Finishing Off

NHS England's Call for Action (General Practice) (2013): http://www.england. nhs.uk/wp-content/uploads/2013/09/igp-cta-evid.pdf

General references and further reading

Ahmad, I., R. Nair, M. Block and G. P. Easton (2014), *How to Pass the CSA Exam: For GP Trainees and MRCGP CSA Candidates*, London: Wiley (ISBN: 978-1118471012).

Booton, P., C. Cooper, G. Easton and M. Harper (2012), *General Practice at a Glance*, Chichester: Wiley-Blackwell (ISBN: 9780470655511).

Curtis, S., N. Tucker, G. Allsopp, K. Fernando and S. Becker (2015), *NB Medical Education Hot Topics GP Update Course*, P&S Medical Education Limited (website: www.nbmedical.com).

Dacre, J. and P. Kopelman (2002), *Handbook of Clinical Skills*, London: Manson Publishing.

'GP Notebook'; www.gpnotebook.co.uk (a concise synopsis of the entire field of clinical medicine focused on the needs of the GP).

Joint Formulary Committee (2015), *British National Formulary* (edition number 70), London: BMJ Group and Pharmaceutical Press.

Moulton, L. (2007), *The Naked Consultation: A Practical Guide to Primary Care Consultation Skills*, Oxford: Radcliffe Publishing.

Websites of health information designed for patients

Patient UK
www.patient.co.uk: Evidence-based information leaflets for patients on a wide range of medical and health topics.

NHS Choices
http://www.nhs.uk/pages/home.aspx: The official website of the National Health Service in England. A comprehensive health information service helping people to make the best choices about their health and lifestyle, but also about making the most of NHS and social care services in England.

Healthtalkonline
www.healthtalkonline.org: Reliable health information from patients, for patients.

Index

313

narratives 10–11, 140–1, 146–7,
 158–9
National Health Service (NHS) 300
National Institute for Health and Care
 Excellence (NICE) guidelines 33,
 71–2, 90, 257–8
nausea 103, 145, 148, 152, 191
neck stiffness 255–6
negligence claims 56
Neighbour, Roger 12–13, 68, 96
noise sensitivity 147
norovirus 263
nystagmus 155, 198

obesity 69
observation 179–80, 219, 264
O'Dowd, Tom 206
oesophageal reflux 17
olive oil drops 129
opening lines 29–30
ophthalmoscope 2, 155–6
opioids 281–5, 304
 withdrawal 282
optic disc 155–6
oral contraceptive pill 62, 148, 152
osteoarthritis 195
otoscope 2
overweight 64, 67–70
overwhelmed, feeling 206, 207–8
oxycodone 280–5
oxygen saturation 124, 268
oxygen therapy 271

paediatricians/paediatrics 249–50,
 257, 272
pain
 abdominal 33, 43, 95, 102–15,
 280, 282–3, 298
 back 95–102, 298
 chest 5–27, 295
 joint 204–7, 214
 and the mind 98–100

muscular 204–7, 214
painkillers 115–16, 280–5, 304
 overuse 142, 153
palpation 20, 21, 112
panic attacks 17
panic buttons 287, 304
papilloedema 155
paracetamol 116, 247, 259
 overdose 91–2
Parkinson's disease 197, 198, 200,
 301
part-time GPs 165, 232
pathology 106
patient health complaint lists
 119–21
Patient Health Questionnaire-9
 (PHQ-9) 85, 92
patient lists 3
patient narratives 10–11, 140–1,
 146–7, 158–9
patient satisfaction scores 56
patient-centred care 14
Patient's Unmet Needs (PUNs) 135
peak expiratory flow rate (PEFR)
 123–4
peak flow meters 123
Pendleton, David 11
penicillin 48, 151, 296
percussion 113–14
performance targets 291
pericarditis 16–17
periods 62, 225, 226–7
peritonism 112
permethrin cream 183, 300
personal illness narratives 140–1,
 146–7, 158–9
personality change 146
petechiae 252–3
phenoxymethylpenicillin 48
phlebotomy 200–1
photophobia (light sensitivity) 147–8,
 152, 256